Allergic Rhinosinusitis and Airway Diseases

Allergic Rhinosinusitis and Airway Diseases

Editor

Sy Duong-Quy

MDPI • Basel • Beijing • Wuhan • Barcelona • Belgrade • Manchester • Tokyo • Cluj • Tianjin

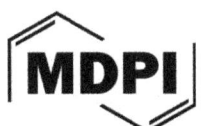

Editor
Sy Duong-Quy
Bio-Medical Research Center
Lam Dong Medical College
Da Lat
Vietnam

Editorial Office
MDPI
St. Alban-Anlage 66
4052 Basel, Switzerland

This is a reprint of articles from the Special Issue published online in the open access journal *Sinusitis* (ISSN 2309-107X) (available at: www.mdpi.com/journal/sinusitis/special_issues/Allergic_Rhino-Sinusitis_and_Airway_Diseases).

For citation purposes, cite each article independently as indicated on the article page online and as indicated below:

LastName, A.A.; LastName, B.B.; LastName, C.C. Article Title. *Journal Name* **Year**, *Volume Number*, Page Range.

ISBN 978-3-0365-4816-6 (Hbk)
ISBN 978-3-0365-4815-9 (PDF)

© 2022 by the authors. Articles in this book are Open Access and distributed under the Creative Commons Attribution (CC BY) license, which allows users to download, copy and build upon published articles, as long as the author and publisher are properly credited, which ensures maximum dissemination and a wider impact of our publications.

The book as a whole is distributed by MDPI under the terms and conditions of the Creative Commons license CC BY-NC-ND.

Contents

About the Editor vii

Preface to "Allergic Rhinosinusitis and Airway Diseases" ix

Sy Duong-Quy
Allergic Rhinosinusitis and Airway Diseases
Reprinted from: *Sinusitis* 2022, 6, 21-25, doi:10.3390/sinusitis6010003 1

Abigail Weaver and Andrew Wood
Promoting Equity When Using the SNOT-22 Score: A Scoping Review and Literature Review
Reprinted from: *Sinusitis* 2022, 6, 15-20, doi:10.3390/sinusitis6010002 7

Snezhina Lazova, Marta Baleva, Stamatios Priftis, Emilia Naseva and Tsvetelina Velikova
Atopic Status in Children with Asthma and Respiratory Allergies—Comparative Analysis of Total IgE, ImmunoCAP Phadiatop/fx5 and Euroimmun Pediatric Immunoblot
Reprinted from: *Sinusitis* 2021, 6, 1-14, doi:10.3390/sinusitis6010001 13

Sy Duong-Quy, Thuy Nguyen-Thi-Dieu, Khai Tran-Quang, Tram Tang-Thi-Thao, Toi Nguyen-Van and Thu Vo-Pham-Minh et al.
Study of Nasal Fractional Exhaled Nitric Oxide (FENO) in Children with Allergic Rhinitis
Reprinted from: *Sinusitis* 2021, 5, 123-131, doi:10.3390/sinusitis5020013 27

Laura Araújo, Vanessa Arata and Ricardo G. Figueiredo
Olfactory Disorders in Post-Acute COVID-19 Syndrome
Reprinted from: *Sinusitis* 2021, 5, 116-122, doi:10.3390/sinusitis5020012 37

Fernando M. Calatayud-Sáez, Blanca Calatayud and Ana Calatayud
Effects of the Traditional Mediterranean Diet in Childhood Recurrent Acute Rhinosinusitis
Reprinted from: *Sinusitis* 2021, 5, 101-115, doi:10.3390/sinusitis5020011 45

Kremena Naydenova, Vasil Dimitrov and Tsvetelina Velikova
Immunological and microRNA Features of Allergic Rhinitis in the Context of United Airway Disease
Reprinted from: *Sinusitis* 2021, 5, 45-52, doi:10.3390/sinusitis5010005 61

Pranav Nair and Kedar Prabhavalkar
Anti-Asthmatic Effects of Saffron Extract and Salbutamol in an Ovalbumin-Induced Airway Model of Allergic Asthma
Reprinted from: *Sinusitis* 2021, 5, 17-31, doi:10.3390/sinusitis5010003 69

Rory Chan, Chris RuiWen Kuo and Brian Lipworth
Low-Grade B Cell Lymphoproliferative Disorder Masquerading as Chronic Rhinosinusitis
Reprinted from: *Sinusitis* 2021, 5, 1-4, doi:10.3390/sinusitis5010001 85

Gyan Chandra Kashyap, Deepanjali Vishwakarma and Shri Kant Singh
Prevalence and Risk Factors of Sinus and Nasal Allergies among Tannery Workers of Kanpur City
Reprinted from: *Sinusitis* 2021, 5, 5-16, doi:10.3390/sinusitis5010002 89

About the Editor

Sy Duong-Quy

Professor Sy Duong-Quy is currently the Director of Lam Dong Medical College and Bio-Medical Research Center. He is also a Professor of Medicine of Penn State University—Division of Immuno-Allergology and Pulmonology; President of Vietnam Society of Sleep Medicine; and Vice-President of Vietnam Respiratory Society. He is an expert in immuno-allergology, respiratory diseases, and sleep medicine. He is also a Fellow of the American College of Chest Physicians (ACCP) and an active member of the American Thoracic Society (ATS), European Respiratory Society (ERS), Asia-Pacific Society of Respirology (APSR), French Language Society of Pulmonology (SPLF), World Sleep Society (WSS) and GINA—GOLD Assembly.

Professor Sy Duong-Quy is a clinical physician who is also very active in both academic teaching and scientific research. He has published more than 140 papers in international journals and book chapters in international textbooks. He is currently the Editor-in-Chief of the *Journal of Functional Ventilation and Pulmonology (JFVP)* and *Journal of Vascular Medicine and Surgery (JVMS)*. He is also an Editorial Board Member of many international peer-reviewed journals.

Preface to "Allergic Rhinosinusitis and Airway Diseases"

The concept of united airway disease interactions comprises allergic rhinosinusitis, including allergic rhinitis, eosinophilic chronic rhinosinusitis, and other upper or lower airway disorders such as obstructive sleep apnea, bronchial hyperresponsiveness and allergic asthma. It embodies a coherent pathophysiology and a comprehensive approach to the treatment of upper and lower airway disorders. The treatment of chronic allergic rhinosinusitis may reduce obstructive sleep apnea symptoms, chronic cough, or the dose of inhaled corticosteroids necessary to treat asthma, and vice versa.

Many objectives in the interaction concept between allergic rhinosinusitis and airway disease management should be achieved in the near future for the reliable control of each disease. More awareness of allergic rhinosinusitis and its comorbidity with other airway diseases must be emphasized in patients' management programs. Progress in diagnosis, with the help of the advanced biomarkers and relevant imagery techniques associated with the accurate treatment of allergic rhinosinusitis and airway diseases, should be developed by scientists to drive the indication and follow-up of target treatment with biologic therapies. Finally, more research on the interaction between allergic rhinosinusitis and airway diseases considered comorbidities or modifiable cofactors should be reconsidered by physicians in the next decade.

This Book covers different interesting topics to give readers an overview of healthcare equality, advanced biomarkers, accurate diagnosis and treatment, occupational exposure-induced upper airway allergy and neoplastic disease mimicking chronic rhinosinusitis.

Sy Duong-Quy
Editor

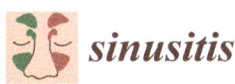

Editorial

Allergic Rhinosinusitis and Airway Diseases

Sy Duong-Quy [1,2,3,4]

1. Clinical Research Unit, Lam Dong Medical College and Bio-Medical Research Center, Dalat 84263, Vietnam; sduongquy.jfvp@gmail.com
2. Consultation Department, Pham Ngoc Thach Medical University, Ho Chi Minh City 8428, Vietnam
3. University Medical Center, Department of Consultation, University of Medicine and Pharmacy at Ho Chi Minh City, Ho Chi Minh City 8428, Vietnam
4. Hershey Medical Center, Division of Pulmonary, Allergy and Critical Care Medicine, Penn State Medical College, Hershey, PA 17033, USA

Citation: Duong-Quy, S. Allergic Rhinosinusitis and Airway Diseases. *Sinusitis* 2022, 6, 21–25. https://doi.org/10.3390/sinusitis6010003

Received: 5 May 2022
Accepted: 12 May 2022
Published: 14 May 2022

Publisher's Note: MDPI stays neutral with regard to jurisdictional claims in published maps and institutional affiliations.

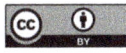

Copyright: © 2022 by the author. Licensee MDPI, Basel, Switzerland. This article is an open access article distributed under the terms and conditions of the Creative Commons Attribution (CC BY) license (https://creativecommons.org/licenses/by/4.0/).

The concept of united airway disease interaction, which comprises chronic rhinosinusitis and other lower airway disorders such as asthma, has been recognized for over a decade. This concept furthers deeper comprehension on the pathophysiology and management of upper and lower airway diseases. In this Special Issue, entitled "Allergic Rhinosinusitis and Airway Diseases", there are nine published papers which cover different interesting topics to give readers an overview of healthcare equality, advanced biomarkers, accurate diagnosis and treatment, occupational exposure-induced upper airway allergy and neoplastic disease mimicking chronic rhinosinusitis.

The equity and equality between races of patients with chronic rhinosinusitis should be considered by physicians. In fact, this issue has previously drawn the attention of the World Health Organization (WHO) [1], and was the focus of a systemic review by Weaver et al. in the Special Issue of *Sinusitis* entitled "Promoting Equity When Using the SNOT-22 Score: A Scoping Review and Literature Review" [2]. In this study, Weaver et al. [2] demonstrated the use of quality-of-life (QoL) tools to assist clinical decision-making by using SNOT-22 in patients with chronic rhinosinusitis to promote equality across diverse populations. The authors emphasized the effects of ethnicity and race on SNOT-22 scores and tried to improve equity. Based on PubMed and MEDLINE searches with appropriate keywords to find papers for a scoping review, Weaver' study revealed, for the first time, that ethnic differences appear to exist in acute sinusitis symptomatology, and ethnic differences also exist with regard to QoL tools. Thus, the authors suggest that the evidence implies that some form of correction to QoL scores could help to promote equity for non-white patients.

Although the main theme of this Special Issue is "*Allergic Rhinosinusitis and Airway Diseases*", currently, the large number of patients who have had the sequelae of COVID-19 within olfactory disorders during the post-COVID-19 phase is also a crucial healthcare problem for ENT (ear–nose–throat) physicians [3]. Therefore, in this Special Issue, Araújo et al. [4] have taken great efforts to successfully summarize the main mechanism and clinical management of anosmia in post-COVID-19 patients. This narrative review describes that olfactory disorder is one of the most common symptoms in patients with acute COVID-19 infection, and most of them recover normal neurosensory function in a short time. However, the authors emphasized that approximately 10% of patients have reported a long-term smell dysfunction which significantly impacts their quality of life. It is clear that inflammation and cellular damage can play a key role in the pathogenesis of olfactory dysfunctions. Based on this pathogenesis, the appropriate management of smell disturbances in post-COVID-19 patients should focus on the underlying mechanisms in combination with adequate smell training.

Recently, the idea of measuring the levels of fractional exhaled nitric oxide (FENO) during the COVID-19 pandemic and in patients with long-COVID has been published [5,6]. This idea might open a new field of research in the use of FENO to screen post-COVID-19 patients with anosmia in clinical practice. Although the measurement of FENO in patients with asthma has been described in recent decades, its use in patients with allergic rhinitis (AR) remains a new area for ENT physicians [7]. In this Special Issue, Duong-Quy et al. have contributed original research on the role of nasal FENO in children with allergic rhinitis [8] to evaluate the correlations between nasal FENO and anthropometric, clinical and functional characteristics, and to determine the cut-off of nasal FENO for diagnosis of AR in the symptomatic children. This study showed that nasal FENO levels in AR patients were significantly higher than control subjects, and nasal FENO was significantly correlated with AR symptoms and nasal inspiratory/expiratory peak flows. Interestingly, the cut-off of nasal FENO for positive AR diagnosis had a very high specificity and sensitivity in AR diagnosis. These authors also concluded that the use of nasal FENO as a biomarker of AR could represent a useful tool and an additional armamentarium in the management of disease (Figure 1).

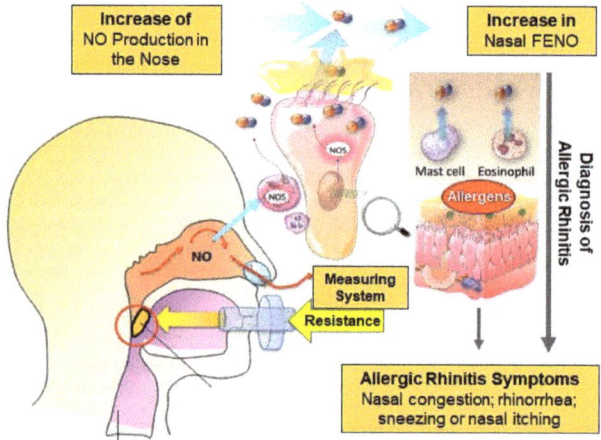

Figure 1. Principle of nasal FENO measurement in subjects with AR. AR: allergic rhinitis; FENO: fractional exhaled nitric oxide; NOS: nitric oxide synthase.

The use of FENO in management of asthma has been approved by many countries and international guidelines [9]; however, nasal FENO has not been approved unanimously in the management of AR. Therefore, other biomarkers used in the management of AR, such as circulating specific non-coding microRNAs (miRNAs), have been presented in another review in this Special Issue: "Allergic Rhinosinusitis and Airway Diseases". This review, entitled *"Immunological and microRNA Features of Allergic Rhinitis in the Context of United Airway Disease"* and written by Naydenova et al. [10], focused on the theory involving inflammation of the upper respiratory tract in patients with AR might contribute to lower respiratory airway inflammation. These authors suggested that T-helper 17 (Th17) cells and related cytokines are also involved in the immunological mechanism of AR along with classical Th2 cells, leading to Th17-induced neutrophilic inflammation in the lungs. Definitely, the regulators of this inflammatory process could be modulated by circulating specific miRNAs, which are distinctively expressed in AR and asthmatic patients. Hence, this pathway could be considered a promising target treatment for the therapy of patients with concomitant AR and asthma.

This Special Issue has been supplemented with the study realized by Nair et al. [11] on the efficacy of saffron extract in an ovalbumin-induced airway model of allergic asthma. This study, using a very-well-known animal model to induce allergic asthma via introducing ovalbumin (OVA) into the nose, again confirmed the unification of the upper and lower airway inflammatory pathways in AR and asthma [12]. In this study, the authors used saffron (*C. sativus*) extract (CSE), a product which exerts anti-inflammatory, anti-allergic and immunomodulatory properties, to investigate its efficacy in combination with salbutamol in the treatment of OVA-induced asthma in rats. The main results of this study demonstrated that the treatment with CSE and salbutamol significantly attenuated OVA-induced Th2 cytokine levels (TNF-α, IL-1β, IL-4, IL-13) in the bloodstream and lung tissue by ameliorating OVA-induced inflammatory influx and ultrastructural aberrations. The authors suggested that the combination of CSE and short-acting beta 2-agonist could be considered a new therapeutic strategy for the management of asthma.

Saffron has been considered as one of the most valuable spices for centuries, and it has been used in daily foods for promoting good health and a positive mood status. Therefore, the results of Nadir's study could develop the current concept related to the use of diet in the treatment of patients with respiratory allergic diseases who did not respond to pharmacological therapy [13]. In the same scope, Calatayud-Sáez et al. [14] have published their results from the study entitled *"Effects of the Traditional Mediterranean Diet in Childhood Recurrent Acute Rhinosinusitis"* in this Special Issue. This study was conducted in a young population (1–5 years old children) who had three or more acute rhinosinusitis episodes in the period of one year from the program *"Learning to Eat from the Mediterranean"* in Spain. The main outcomes of this study showed that more than 50% of study subjects did not have any episode of acute rhinosinusitis, and KIDMED (Mediterranean Diet Quality Index) scores increased significantly. These authors stated that adoption of the traditional Mediterranean diet might have a promising effect on the prevention and treatment of recurrent acute and chronic rhinosinusitis in early ages of life.

An appropriate diet, such as the traditional Mediterranean diet, may be useful for subjects who are allergic with airborne and/or food allergens. For these subjects, skin prick tests (SPT) have been considered as a relevant examination technique to detect respiratory or food allergens, although the level of specificity remains a challenge for the treatment with specific desensibilization [15]. Therefore, the atopic status assessment with SPT or specific immunoglobulin (sIgE) in subjects with asthma or AR is always a milestone in identifying potential risk factors and triggers provoking loss of disease control. A recent study in asthmatic children published by Lazova et al. [16] demonstrated that there was a moderate to strong correlation between multiscreen ImmunoCAP Phadiatop/fx5 and Euroimmun sIgE titers against aero-allergens—cats, mites, tree mix and food allergens—soy, wheat, rice, apple and peanut. This study also showed that good sensitivity and specificity were observed for EUROIMMUN Pediatric (food allergens) compared with the gold standard ImmunoCap/fx5. The authors of this study suggested that the immunoblotting technique is an easily applicable, cost-effective and reliable alternative to ImmunoCAP Phadiatop/fx5 in diagnosing atopic children.

In addition to airborne and food allergens, some evaporated chemical products used in industry could be the cause of airway allergies in workers [17]. This crucial problem has been clarified by the study realized by Kashyap et al., published in this Special Issue of *Sinusitis* [18]. This study included tannery workers of Kanpur city in India who were frequently exposed to chromium during the leather tanning process. The authors found that the severity of nasal and sinus allergies increased with age and work duration in the tannery, and workers with occupational exposure were more likely to develop sinus problems than those without exposure. The authors suggest that this high risk of occupational factors could be eliminated by improving the overall working conditions and ensuring necessary protective regulations for the tannery workers to reduce upper airway allergies and other carcinogenic factors.

This Special Issue, "Allergic Rhinosinusitis and Airway Diseases", concludes with the ninth paper presenting an interesting clinical case, entitled *"Low-Grade B Cell Lymphoproliferative Disorder Masquerading as Chronic Rhinosinusitis"*, reported by Chen et al. [19]. In this case report, a 72-year-old man was referred by his general practitioner for symptoms mimicking chronic rhinosinusitis unresponsive to local corticosteroid treatment and antibiotics. Although the histopathology result taken from the middle turbinate biopsy revealed chronic non-specific inflammatory changes with mixed microbial flora, the patient was consequently referred to hematology specialists, as recommended previously [20]. Then, a combination of serum and radiological findings (chest CT scan: mediastinal and hilar lymphadenopathy; Figure 2) was used to perform the clinical diagnosis of B-cell lymphoproliferative disorder. The authors of this case report recommend that patients with chronic rhinosinusitis who present with atypical clinical features such as nasal crusting and treatment resistant organisms may have underlying immunosuppression.

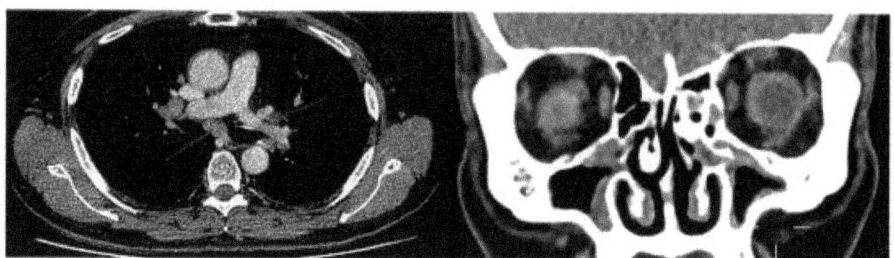

Figure 2. Transverse CT chest image with arrows indicating mediastinal and hilar lymphadenopathy. Coronal CT sinus image depicting disease affecting the ethmoid bullae and ostio-meatal complex [19].

In conclusion, this Special Issue, entitled "Allergic Rhinosinusitis and Airway Diseases", successfully raises more awareness of rhinosinusitis and its comorbidity with other airway diseases. Hence, the concept of united airway disease interaction comprising upper and lower airway diseases should be recognized in patient management programs. Progress in diagnosis, with the use of the advanced biomarkers and relevant imagery techniques associated with accurate treatment of chronic rhinosinusitis and lower airway diseases, should continue to be developed in the future.

Funding: This research received no external funding.

Conflicts of Interest: The author declares no conflict of interest.

References

1. Available online: https://www.who.int/data/health-equity (accessed on 2 May 2022).
2. Weaver, A.; Wood, A. Promoting Equity When Using the SNOT-22 Score: A Scoping Review and Literature Review. *Sinusitis* **2022**, *6*, 15–20. [CrossRef]
3. Algahtani, S.N.; Alzarroug, A.F.; Alghamdi, H.K.; Algahtani, H.K.; Alsywina, N.B.; Bin Abdulrahman, K.A. Investigation on the Factors Associated with the Persistence of Anosmia and Ageusia in Saudi COVID-19 Patients. *Int. J. Environ. Res. Public Health* **2022**, *19*, 1047. [CrossRef] [PubMed]
4. Araújo, L.; Arata, V.; Figueiredo, R.G. Olfactory Disorders in Post-Acute COVID-19 Syndrome. *Sinusitis* **2021**, *5*, 116–122. [CrossRef]
5. Duong-Quy, S.; Ngo-Minh, X.; Tang-Le-Quynh, T.; Tang-Thi-Thao, T.; Nguyen-Quoc, B.; Le-Quang, K.; Tran-Thanh, D.; Doan-Thi-Quynh, N.; Canty, E.; Do, T.; et al. The use of exhaled nitric oxide and peak expiratory flow to demonstrate improved breathability and antimicrobial properties of novel face mask made with sustainable filter paper and Folium Plectranthii amboinicii oil: Additional option for mask shortage during COVID-19 pandemic. *Multidiscip. Respir. Med.* **2020**, *15*, 664. [PubMed]
6. Hua-Huy, T.; Lorut, C.; Aubourg, F.; Morbieu, C.; Marey, J.; Texereau, J.; Fajac, I.; Mouthon, L.; Roche, N.; Dinh-Xuan, A.T. Persistent nasal inflammation 5 months after acute anosmia in patients with COVID-19. *Am. J. Respir. Crit. Care Med.* **2021**, *203*, 1319–1322. [CrossRef] [PubMed]
7. Duong-Quy, S. Clinical utility of the exhaled nitric oxide (NO) measurement with portable devices in the management of allergic airway inflammation and asthma. *J. Asthma Allergy* **2019**, *12*, 331–341. [CrossRef] [PubMed]
8. Duong-Quy, S.; Nguyen-Thi-Dieu, T.; Tran-Quang, K.; Tang-Thi-Thao, T.; Nguyen-Van, T.; Vo-Pham-Minh, T.; Vu-Tran-Thien, Q.; Bui-Diem, K.; Nguyen-Nhu, V.; Hoang-Thi, L.; et al. Study of nasal fractional exhaled nitric oxide (FENO) in children with allergic rhinitis. *Sinusitis* **2021**, *5*, 123–131. [CrossRef]
9. Global Initiative for Asthma. Archived Reports. Available online: http://ginasthma.org/archived-reports/ (accessed on 26 April 2022).
10. Naydenova, K.; Dimitrov, V.; Velikova, T. Immunological and microRNA Features of Allergic Rhinitis in the Context of United Airway Disease. *Sinusitis* **2021**, *5*, 45–52. [CrossRef]

11. Nair, P.; Prabhavalkar, K. Anti-Asthmatic Effects of Saffron Extract and Salbutamol in an Ovalbumin-Induced Airway Model of Allergic Asthma. *Sinusitis* **2021**, *5*, 17–31. [CrossRef]
12. Duong-Quy, S.; Vu-Minh, T.; Hua-Huy, T.; Tang-Thi-Thao, T.; Le-Quang, K.; Tran-Thanh, D.; Doan-Thi-Quynh, N.; Le-Dong, N.N.; Craig, T.J.; Dinh-Xuan, A.T. Study of nasal exhaled nitric oxide levels in diagnosis of allergic rhinitis in subjects with and without asthma. *J. Asthma Allergy* **2017**, *10*, 75–82. [CrossRef] [PubMed]
13. Calatayud-Sáez, F.M.; Calatayud, B.; Luque, M.; Calatayud, A.; Gallego, J.G.; Rivas-Ruiz, F. Effects of the affinity to the Mediterranean diet pattern together with breastfeeding on the incidence of childhood asthma and other inflammatory and recurrent diseases. *Allergol. Et Immunopathol.* **2021**, *49*, 48–55. [CrossRef] [PubMed]
14. Calatayud-Sáez, F.M.; Calatayud, B.; Calatayud, A. Effects of the Traditional Mediterranean Diet in Childhood Recurrent Acute Rhinosinusitis. *Sinusitis* **2021**, *5*, 101–115. [CrossRef]
15. Nevis, I.F.; Binkley, K.; Kabali, C. Diagnostic accuracy of skin-prick testing for allergic rhinitis: A systematic review and meta-analysis. *Allergy Asthma Clin. Immunol.* **2016**, *12*, 20. [CrossRef] [PubMed]
16. Lazova, S.; Baleva, M.; Priftis, S.; Naseva, E.; Velikova, T. Atopic Status in Children with Asthma and Respiratory Allergies-Comparative Analysis of Total IgE, ImmunoCAP Phadiatop/fx5 and Euroimmun Pediatric Immunoblot. *Sinusitis* **2022**, *6*, 1–14. [CrossRef]
17. da Paz, E.R.; de Lima, C.M.F.; Felix, S.N.; Schaeffer, B.; Galvão, C.E.S.; Correia, A.T.; Righetti, R.F.; de Arruda Martins, M.; de Fátima Lopes Calvo Tibério, I.; Saraiva-Romanholo, B.M. Airway inflammatory profile among cleaning workers from different workplaces. *BMC Pulm Med.* **2020**, *22*, 170. [CrossRef] [PubMed]
18. Kashyap, G.C.; Vishwakarma, D.; Singh, S.K. Prevalence and Risk Factors of Sinus and Nasal Allergies among Tannery Workers of Kanpur City. *Sinusitis* **2021**, *5*, 5–16. [CrossRef]
19. Chan, R.; Kuo, C.R.; Lipworth, B. Low-Grade B Cell Lymphoproliferative Disorder Masquerading as Chronic Rhinosinusitis. *Sinusitis* **2021**, *5*, 1–4. [CrossRef]
20. Debord, C.; Wuillème, S.; Eveillard, M.; Theisen, O.; Godon, C.; Le Bris, Y.; Béné, M.C. Flow cytometry in the diagnosis of mature B-cell lymphoproliferative disorders. *Int. J. Lab. Hematol.* **2020**, *42*, 113–120. [CrossRef] [PubMed]

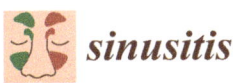

Review

Promoting Equity When Using the SNOT-22 Score: A Scoping Review and Literature Review

Abigail Weaver [1,2] and Andrew Wood [2,3,4,*]

1. Hawkes Bay District Health Board, Hastings 4120, New Zealand; abigail.weaver@hbdhb.govt.nz
2. Waikato Institute of Surgical Education and Research, Hamilton 3204, New Zealand
3. Waikato Clinical Campus, The University of Auckland, Hamilton 3204, New Zealand
4. Department of Otolaryngology, Waikato District Health Board, Hamilton 3204, New Zealand
* Correspondence: andrew.wood@auckland.ac.nz; Tel.: +64-(0)7-839-8750; Fax: +64-(0)7-839-8712

Abstract: It is established that non-white people experience worse health outcomes than white people within the same population. Equity addresses differences between patient subgroups, allowing needs-based distribution of resources. The use of quality-of-life (QoL) tools to assist clinical decision making such as the SNOT-22 for chronic rhinosinusitis promotes equality, not equity, as quality-of-life (QoL) tools provide the same criteria of symptom scoring across diverse populations. We considered the effects of ethnicity and race on SNOT-22 scores and whether these scores should be adjusted to improve equity. PubMed and MEDLINE provided papers for a scoping review. A combination of the following search terms was used: patient-reported outcome measures (PROM) (OR) quality of life; (AND) race (OR) ethnicity (OR) disparities; (AND) otolaryngology (OR) SNOT-22 (OR) sinusitis. The first study identified no evidence of ethnic variability in SNOT-22 scores. However, the study did not represent the local population, including 86% white people. Other studies identified baseline SNOT-22 disparities with respect to population demographics, gender, and age. Ethnic differences appear to exist in acute sinusitis symptomatology. In other fields both within and outside of otorhinolaryngology, ethnic differences exist with regard to QoL tools. This scoping review identified a paucity of data in rhinology. However, evidence implies some form of correction to QoL scores could help promote equity for non-white patients.

Keywords: otolaryngology; sinusitis; ethnic groups; patient-reported outcome measures; quality of life; social justice

1. Introduction

The importance of equity is increasingly recognized and discussed within healthcare generally and within rhinology in particular [1]. Equity in healthcare is defined as "the absence of avoidable or remediable differences among groups of people, whether those groups are defined socially, economically, demographically, or geographically" [2]. The World Health Organization (WHO) explains equity as overcoming and avoiding disparities that infringe on justice and fairness. While equity and equality both target fairness, equality is based on the equal distribution of a commodity within a population, whereas equity is based on unequal distribution to accommodate for differences in need. Therefore, they are fundamentally different principles, potentially at odds with each other. The use of quality-of-life (QoL) tools to facilitate clinical decision making promotes equality, i.e., treating everyone the same. However, if QoL tools do not sufficiently represent different patient groups, their use may prove a potential impediment to equity.

While noting that race and ethnicity are related terms, one's race is the inherited phenotypic attribute of a person. In contrast, one's ethnicity relates to the cultural factors, from a particular group, with which an individual identifies [3].

We have identified, within our New Zealand population, that non-white, minority ethnicities are underrepresented in Public Hospital Rhinology clinics and operating lists [4,5].

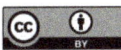

This is despite data indicating that non-white populations appear to have a higher burden of rhinologic diseases. While the reasons for this are likely to be multi-factorial [4], we aimed to consider whether the processes that we as rhinologists use, might be contributing to this apparent inequity, and if so, how this might be addressed.

Chronic rhinosinusitis (CRS) is a non-fatal condition, the treatment of which is directed toward managing symptoms [6]. The ability to quantify symptoms through QoL tools is, therefore, of great importance in CRS management and decision making with regard to appropriate treatment options. The WHO defines QoL as "the individual's perception of their position in life in the context of the culture and value systems in which they live and in relation to their goals" [7]. With regard to the assessment of QoL in CRS, the 22-item Sinonasal Outcome Test (SNOT-22) has become the sentinel subjective assessment of disease severity [8], with 3560 articles returned on a Google Scholar search of "SNOT-22" (search performed 4 April 2021).

Given the importance of the SNOT-22 score in surgical decision making for CRS patients and apparent inequities in the provision of treatment, we wished to investigate the effects of race and ethnicity on the SNOT-22 QoL tool and whether the total SNOT-22 score should be adjusted for patient race or ethnicity when used for clinical decision making. We hypothesize that in the context of comparable disease burden, non-white groups record lower total SNOT-22 scores.

2. Methods

A scoping review technique found peer-reviewed journal papers that met the following inclusion criteria: (1) published between 2010 and 2021; (2) written in English; (3) involved preoperative symptom reporting; (4) provided details of patient demographic; (5) specifically discussed the impact of demographic on symptom scoring in otorhinolaryngology diseases. The following bibliographic databases identified relevant documents from 2010 to 2021: MEDLINE and PubMed. Exclusion criteria included (1) studies published before 2010; (2) papers without English translation; (3) papers that did not compare demographic disparities on symptom scores in otorhinolaryngology disease. The initial search occurred in January 2021 and was repeated in August 2021 to ensure new relevant data were included. The below search strategy was created by one reviewer in collaboration with the Waikato Clinical Campus Librarian. The studies were identified using the selection criteria above.

Search Terms:
1. Patient-reported outcome measures (PROM) (OR) quality of life;
2. (AND) race (OR) ethnicity (OR) disparities;
3. (AND) otolaryngology (OR) SNOT-22 (OR) sinusitis.

The search was followed by analyzing the title, abstract, and subject headings to identify papers that met the study criteria. Reference lists of the identified papers were scanned for similar articles, generating a further literature review. Two reviewers determined the relevance of the studies prior to inclusion into the study. To prevent biased studies influencing data outcomes, the demographics of the studies' local population were compared with the study populations. Reference number five was included as a local preprint publication.

3. Results

Following the method, PubMed identified 1444 papers without using the quality-of-life search term, and MEDLINE/OVID identified 30 papers from the above search.

There was a paucity within the literature explicitly related to PROMs and ethnic/race disparities, and even fewer for the SNOT-22 specifically. A publication on chronic rhinosinusitis identified that less than 10% of American studies provided information on minority-specific demographics when discussing ESS surgical outcomes. It also identified minority populations made up less than half the national census estimates receiving ESS [9].

(1) Results discussing ethnicity/race SNOT22 scores at the time of diagnosis of CRS

One relevant study, at a tertiary rhinology clinic in Boston, Massachusetts, indeed discussed influences of the recruited population demographics. The conclusion was made that there was no evidence identified of disparity between ethnic and racial groupings to their SNOT-22 scores. The population included 300 adult patients with CRS. The study analyzed the patients' symptom scores (SNOT-22 and EuroQol 5-dimensional visual analog scale), age, race, ethnicity, smoking status, medication usage, and comorbidities. The racial groupings for the study cohort were classified as "white" (281 patients), "Black or African American" (5 patients), or "other" (14 patients). The ethnicity groupings were classified as "non-Hispanic" (246 patients), "Hispanic" (9 patients), and "declined to respond" (45 patients). The relatively small groups meant the confidence intervals were large (and therefore reported no statistically significant difference). However, on multivariate analysis, "non-white and/or Hispanic" patients recorded a SNOT-22 score of −2.2 (−11.5 to 7.0), compared with "white, non-Hispanic" patients [10].

Further studies identified within the scoping review attempted to compare disparities in SNOT-22 scores for race and ethnicity, indicating that minority populations have increased SNOT-22 scores at the time of CRS diagnosis. Kuhar et al. (2019) reported that African American patients had higher SNOT-22 scores, compared with white patients (50.7 vs. 1.5, $p < 0.022$). It was also noted, however, that histologic measures of disease severity including eosinophils per high power field, polypoidal disease, subepithelial disease, hyperplastic/papillary changes, and fibrosis indicated a more significant disease burden within the African American population [11]. Similarly, the same pattern of increased SNOT-22 scores at the time of diagnosis was described in Hispanic patients, compared with non-Hispanic patients (55 vs. 37, $p < 0.001$), by Levine et al. (2021). Hispanics, however, also had objective evidence of more severe CRS, such as the presence of nasal polyps (RR = 2.5; 95% CI: 1.0–5.9), neo-osteogenesis, extended procedures, and tissue eosinophilia [12].

(2) Demographic disparities identified in SNOT22 score—not related to ethnicity/race

A cross-sectional study in Brazil identified disparities in SNOT-22 scores for gender and age. Although these are disparities within the same ethnicity and race, this study implies that differences between subgroups may impact PROMS, irrespective of disease severity. There was a statistically significant ($p = 0.005$) difference of two points in the baseline SNOT-22 scores between genders. Men without CRS had a baseline SNOT-22 score of 7, compared with women, whose baseline score was 9. Age over 60 years also indicated a significantly lower score of 7, compared with the younger age groups scores of 8–10 [13].

(3) Ethnic variability in sinonasal symptoms

The same group in Boston has studied ethnic disparities in symptomatology and presentation in the context of acute rhinosinusitis (ARS). They performed a retrospective study of 1,632,826 visits to hospital emergency departments (EDs) where ARS was diagnosed. Compared with white patients, Black ($p = 0.038$) and Hispanic patients ($p = 0.019$) presenting to EDs were less likely to complain of typical sinonasal symptoms. Hispanic patients also reported less typical ARS symptoms such as cough, sputum production, head cold, or flu-like symptoms [14].

(4) Ethnic variation in symptom reporting in otorhinolaryngology

The literature review identified that within other otorhinolaryngology (ORL) fields, studies have identified ethnic disparities in the self-reporting of symptoms. For example, in a study of 5236 women of child-bearing age, the objective measure of hours slept was compared with self-reported trouble sleeping. Women from minorities experienced fewer nights of adequate sleep than white women. However, white women had statistically significantly increased odds of reporting trouble sleeping than minority populations, with an adjusted odds ratio (OR) of 0.47 and 0.29, compared with Black and Hispanic women, respectively. This is still evident when controlling for hours slept [15].

Ethnic/racial disparities in patient-reported outcome measures have also been noted in laryngology. After controlling for influential demographics including education, income, and health insurance, minorities' self-reported voice problems had decreased OR, compared with white Americans, with African Americans reporting an OR of 0.83 and Hispanics 0.63 and remaining minorities at 0.69, compared with white adults [16].

(5) Ethnic variation in symptom reporting outside of otorhinolaryngology

There are ethnic inequities in symptom reporting and QoL surveys in multiple medical fields, for instance, in HIV symptom management. The literature review identified Black non-Hispanics were significantly underreporting "fatigue, depression, muscle aches, anxiety, difficulties with memory and concentration" with compared to other ethnicities [17].

4. Discussion

It is essential to identify limitations in QoL measures with regard to whether they contribute to current health inequities. If our hypothesis is correct that minorities with CRS are under-reporting symptoms on SNOT-22 surveys, white people may be preferentially prioritized for intervention over minority populations, thus contributing to health disparities that unjustly harm minority populations. Although not directly addressing our question around race and ethnicity, it has been identified that different groups within society do report different mean SNOT-22 scores [13].

It is well established that some non-whites suffer worse health outcomes than white people. In our New Zealand population, many studies have shown worse health outcomes for the indigenous Māori population, compared with non-Māori. In a literature review, a study was identified in which Māori was significantly less likely to be offered chemotherapy than non-Māori and was more likely to experience delays within the first eight weeks before chemotherapy. Another study discussed in this review found Māori women were significantly less likely to receive pain relief during labor; furthermore, doctors of European ethnicity spent 17 % less time with Māori patients than other ethnic groups [18]. Recent studies in our department demonstrated a significant under-representation of minority ethnicities in rhinology clinics and operating theatres [4]. The reasons for such ethnic disparities are likely multi-factorial [4] but may include that disease burden in non-white populations is relatively under-represented when QoL is quantified.

US minority populations also experience similar inequities. The National Health Interview Survey identified that white adults with CRS had an increased likelihood of receiving specialist appointments and intervention than minority populations [9]. A retrospective study of 1344 adults with CRS showed that African Americans who underwent operations showed greater objective severity of refractory CRS [19]. Another study of 4337 patients identified that African Americans and Hispanic patients had higher requirements for urgent operations for sinusitis ($p = 0.003$ and $p < 0.001$, respectively) [20], presumably representing lower access to elective care.

Our scoping review highlighted a paucity of data regarding the effect of race and ethnicity on SNOT-22 scores. Although the Bergmark (2018) study was commendable in its intentions, this data had significant limitations. First, considering racial groupings, 93.7% of the study population identified as white, in a city where recent census data show that 44.4% are white [21]. This implies a high risk of selection bias. Although some power calculations were performed, ethnicity and racial groupings of the size reported would appear liable to a type 2 error, noting that a non-significant trend toward lower QoL scores was reported in non-white patients. Finally, the groupings assessed—namely, white vs. non-white and Hispanic vs. non-Hispanic, cannot be considered generalizable to all ethnic and racial groupings. Based on this one study, and noting its limitations, it seems inappropriate, therefore, to generalize that ethnicity does not impact total SNOT-22 scores.

Two articles report higher total SNOT-22 scores within minority populations at presentation. However, they also identify that the disease burden was substantially higher in those groups. Thus, the comparison of SNOT-22 scores does not identify if minority populations with equivalent CRS severity under-report on total SNOT-22 scores [11,12].

Data from other fields both within and outside of ORL indicate that ethnic variabilities exist regarding self-reporting of symptom burden with symptoms relatively under-represented by non-white populations. It seems reasonable to hypothesize, therefore, that using the SNOT-22 score or other QoL measures in rhinology contributes to inequitable treatment of non-white populations. Unfortunately, however, we are unable to prove or disprove this hypothesis.

The described study of ARS patients may be limited by an inaccurate diagnosis of ARS in the ED setting, owing to differential diagnoses such as migraine. However, it does raise the possibility that there may be ethnic and racial variation within the various SNOT-22 domains, as well as with respect to the total SNOT-22 score, meriting further study.

In summary, the literature discussed in this review identifies ethnic variability in symptom reporting. However, there are no conclusive data to prove or disprove our hypothesis. Research is required to identify ethnic variations in total SNOT-22 scores but also within the domains of the SNOT-22 score. Ideally, a large prospective study with ethnic and racial groupings representative of the local population should be performed. This would ideally be a multi-centered or even multi-national study. This study may face challenges owing to the inadequate referral of non-white patients to tertiary centers, generating selection bias. Objective measures such as the Lund-Mackay score (LMS) or endoscopic scores could be used as comparators.

5. Conclusions

While our scoping review has indicated a paucity of data in rhinology related to ethnicity and QoL tools/PROMS, evidence from other population subgroups and fields of medicine cast doubt on the effectiveness of the SNOT-22 tool to assess the severity of CRS equitably in non-white populations. Without the use of a correction, the use of QoL tools such as the SNOT-22 may contribute to white patients preferentially being offered intervention. In the pursuit of more equitable practice, further study is merited in this field.

Author Contributions: Conceptualization, A.W. (Andrew Wood); methodology, A.W. (Abigail Weaver); validation, A.W. (Andrew Wood) and A.W. (Abigail Weaver); data curation, A.W. (Abigail Weaver); writing—original draft preparation, A.W. (Abigail Weaver) and A.W. (Andrew Wood); writing—review and editing, A.W. (Andrew Wood); visualization, A.W. (Abigail Weaver); supervision, A.W. (Andrew Wood). All authors have read and agreed to the published version of the manuscript.

Funding: This research received no external funding.

Institutional Review Board Statement: Not applicable.

Informed Consent Statement: Not applicable.

Data Availability Statement: Data are available through MEDLINE and PubMed using the references below.

Conflicts of Interest: The authors declare no conflict of interest.

References

1. Gray, S.; Wise, S.; Welch, K.; Bleier, B.; Kern, R.; Lin, S.; Luong, A.; Schlosser, R.; Soler, Z.; Turner, J. Editorial: Valuing diversity, equity and inclusion. *Int. Forum Allergy Rhinol.* **2021**, *11*, 5. [CrossRef] [PubMed]
2. WHO. Equity. Who.Int. 2020. Available online: https://www.who.int/healthsystems/topics/equity/en/ (accessed on 25 December 2020).
3. Eriksen, T. *Ethnicity and Nationalism*; Pluto Press: Sterling, VA, USA, 2015. [CrossRef]
4. Cate, L.; van der Werf, B.; Wood, A. The complexities of practising equitable Rhinology within resource limitations. *Aust. J. Otolaryngol.* **2021**, *4*, 22. [CrossRef]
5. Ratnayake Kumar, A.; Wood, A.J. Equity, deprivation and access to endoscopic sinus surgery in the Waikato region of New Zealand. *ANZ J. Surg-Preprint*, 2021; submitted.
6. Fokkens, W.J.; Lund, V.J.; Hopkins, C.; Hellings, P.W.; Kern, R.; Reitsma, S.; Toppila-Salmi, S.; Bernal-Sprekelsen, M.; Mullol, J.; Alobid, I.; et al. European Position Paper on Rhinosinusitis and Nasal Polyps 2020. *Rhinology* **2020**, *58*, 1–464. [CrossRef] [PubMed]

7. The World Health Organization. WHOQOL—Measuring Quality of Life. Who.Int. 2020. Available online: https://www.who.int/tools/whoqol#:~{}:text=WHO%20defines%20Quality%20of%20Life,%2C%20expectations%2C%20standards%20and%20concerns (accessed on 25 December 2020).
8. Beswick, D.; Mace, J.; Soler, Z.; Ayoub, N.F.; Rudmik, L.; DeCondem, A.S.; Smith, T.L. Appropriateness criteria predict outcomes for sinus surgery and may aid in future patient selection. *Laryngoscope* **2018**, *128*, 2448–2454. [CrossRef] [PubMed]
9. Soler, Z.; Mace, J.; Litvack, J.; Smith, T. Chronic Rhinosinusitis, Race, and Ethnicity. *Am. J. Rhinol. Allergy* **2012**, *26*, 110–116. [CrossRef] [PubMed]
10. Bergmark, R.W.; Hoehle, L.P.; Chyou, D.; Phillips, K.M.; Caradonna, D.S.; Gray, S.T.; Sedaghat, A.R. Association of Socioeconomic Status, Race and Insurance Status with Chronic Rhinosinusitis Patient-Reported Outcome Measures. *Otolaryngol.—Head Neck Surg.* **2018**, *158*, 571–579. [CrossRef] [PubMed]
11. Kuhar, H.N.; Ganti, A.; Eggerstedt, M.; Mahdavinia, M.; Gattuso, P.; Ghai, R.; Batra, P.S.; Tajudeen, B.A. The impact of race and insurance status on baseline histopathology profile in patients with chronic rhinosinusitis. *Int. Forum. Allergy Rhinol.* **2019**, *9*, 665–673. [CrossRef] [PubMed]
12. Levine, C.; Casiano, R.; Lee, D.; Mantero, A.; Liu, X.; Palacio, A. Chronic Rhinosinusitis Disease Disparity in the South Florida Hispanic Population. *Laryngoscope* **2021**, *131*, 2659–2665. [CrossRef] [PubMed]
13. Gregório, L.L.; Andrade, J.S.; Caparroz, F.A.; Saraceni Neto, P.; Kosugi, E.M. Influence of age and gender in the normal values of Sino Nasal Outcome Test-22. *Clin. Otolaryngol.* **2015**, *40*, 115–120. [CrossRef] [PubMed]
14. Bergmark, R.W.; Sedaghat, A.R. Presentation to Emergency Departments for Acute Rhinosinusitis: Disparities in Symptoms by Race and Insurance Status. *Otolaryngol.—Head Neck Surg.* **2016**, *155*, 790–796. [CrossRef] [PubMed]
15. Amyx, M.; Xiong, X.; Xie, Y.; Buekens, P. Racial/Ethnic Differences in Sleep Disorders and Reporting of Trouble Sleeping among Women of Childbearing Age in the United States. *Matern. Child Health J.* **2017**, *21*, 306–314. [CrossRef] [PubMed]
16. Hur, K.; Zhou, S.; Bertelsen, C.; Johns, M.M., 3rd. Health disparities among adults with voice problems in the United States. *Laryngoscope* **2018**, *128*, 915–920. [CrossRef] [PubMed]
17. Schnall, R.; Siegel, K.; Jia, H.; Olender, S.; Hirshfield, S. Racial and socioeconomic disparities in the symptom reporting of persons living with HIV. *AIDS Care* **2018**, *30*, 774–783. [CrossRef] [PubMed]
18. Houkamau, C. What you can't see can hurt you: How do stereotyping, implicit bias and stereotype threat affect Maori health? *MAI J. N. Z. J. Indig. Scholarsh.* **2016**, *5*, 124–136. [CrossRef]
19. Mahdavinia, M.; Benhammuda, M.; Codispoti, C.D.; Tobin, M.C.; Losavio, P.S.; Mehta, A.; Jeffe, J.S.; Bandi, S.; Peters, A.T.; Stevens, W.W.; et al. African American Patients with Chronic Rhinosinusitis Have a Distinct Phenotype of Polyposis Associated with Increased Asthma Hospitalization. *J. Allergy Clin. Immunol. Pract.* **2016**, *4*, 658–664.e1. [CrossRef] [PubMed]
20. Pecha, P.P.; Hamberis, A.; Patel, T.A.; Melvin, C.L.; Ford, M.E.; Andrews, A.L.; White, D.R.; Schlosser, R.J. Racial Disparities in Pediatric Endoscopic Sinus Surgery. *Laryngoscope* **2021**, *131*, E1369–E1374. [CrossRef] [PubMed]
21. Boston, MA. Data USA. Datausa.io. 2020. Available online: https://datausa.io/profile/geo/boston-ma/#demographics (accessed on 25 December 2020).

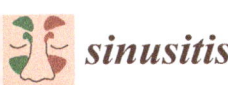 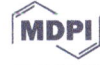

Article

Atopic Status in Children with Asthma and Respiratory Allergies—Comparative Analysis of Total IgE, ImmunoCAP Phadiatop/fx5 and Euroimmun Pediatric Immunoblot

Snezhina Lazova [1,2,*], Marta Baleva [3], Stamatios Priftis [4], Emilia Naseva [5] and Tsvetelina Velikova [6]

1. Pediatric Department, University Hospital N. I. Pirogov, 1606 Sofia, Bulgaria
2. Healthcare Department, Faculty of Public Health "Prof. Tsekomir Vodenicharov, MD, DSc", Medical University Sofia, 1431 Sofia, Bulgaria
3. Clinic of Clinical Immunology and Stem Cell Bank, University Hospital Alexandrovska, 1431 Sofia, Bulgaria; marta_baleva@yahoo.com
4. Department of Health Technology Assessment, Faculty of Public Health "Prof. Tsekomir Vodenicharov, MD, DSc", Medical University of Sofia, 1527 Sofia, Bulgaria; stamatios.priftis@gmail.com
5. Department of Health Economics, Faculty of Public Health "Prof. Tsekomir Vodenicharov, MD, DSc", Medical University of Sofia, 1527 Sofia, Bulgaria; emilia.naseva@gmail.com
6. Department of Clinical Immunology, University Hospital Lozenetsz, Sofia University, 1407 Sofia, Bulgaria; ts_velikova@abv.bg
* Correspondence: snejina@lazova.com

Abstract: Introduction: An atopic status assessment (skin prick test or specific immunoglobulin (sIgE)) in asthmatic children is considered a milestone in identifying potential risk factors and triggers provoking loss of asthma control and asthma exacerbation. Objective: The study aims to perform a comparative analysis of different laboratory methods for a serological assessment of an atopic status in asthma and respiratory allergies in children. Material and methods: A total of 86 children were included, all of whom were diagnosed with bronchial asthma, aged from 5 to 17 years and screened for total IgE level using enzyme-linked immunosorbent assay (ELISA). In 48 randomly selected children, we performed a semi-quantitative serological in vitro assessment of the specific IgE antibodies against food and aeroallergen, using two different laboratory methods—Euroimmun Immunoblot and ImmunoCAP (Phadiatop/fx5). Results: In 70% of the children with a history of allergies, and 65.3% without clinically manifested allergies, multiscreen test ImmunoCAP Phadiatop/fx5 showed positivity and confirmed atopy. Our results showed a significant moderate to strong correlation between multiscreen ImmunoCAP Phadiatop/fx5, and Euroimmun specific IgE titers against aeroallergens—cats, mites, tree mix and food allergens—soy, wheat (= 0.006), rice, = 0.090), apple = 0.007) and peanut. A sensitivity of 63% and specificity of 73.5% was observed for EUROIMMUN Pediatric (food allergens, IgE titer > 1) compared with the gold standard ImmunoCap/fx5. The mean value of total IgE is significantly higher in children with asthma and concomitant with allergic rhinitis compared to those without allergic rhinitis (mean 202.52 U/mL, IQR 102.50 (24.20–363.95) vs. 316.68, IQR 261.00 (109.20–552.50), $p = 0.005$). Conclusion: Establishing the spectrum of the most common respiratory and food allergens is an essential factor for maintaining asthma control, both through a strategy to avoid allergen exposure and by developing a recommendation plan. The immunoblotting technique is easily applicable in daily clinical and laboratory practice. It is also a cost-effective and reliable alternative to the "gold standard" ImmunoCAP Phadiatop/fx5 in diagnosing atopy in children.

Keywords: atopic status; allergic rhinitis; total IgE; specific IgE; childhood asthma; immunoblot; ImmunoCAP

1. Introduction

In epidemiological studies, atopy and allergy have been associated as risk factors for bronchial hyperreactivity and asthma in children and adults [1,2]. Atopy is defined as a tendency to produce IgE antibodies in response to allergen exposure. This increases the risk of developing diseases such as asthma, allergic rhinitis (AR) or atopic dermatitis (AD) [3]. Atopy can range from asymptomatic sensitization to one or more allergens with no clinical presentation to clinically manifested atopic disease. During childhood, sensitization is predominantly an immunological phenomenon [4,5]. In clinical practice, atopy is often equated with the presence of serum allergen-specific IgE antibodies or positive skin prick test (SPT). However, a positive SPT is not always associated with clinical manifestations of established sensitization. In fact, some "atopic" children do not develop any allergic diseases [6]. Skin allergy testing is generally more sensitive than in vitro studies [6]. However, serum-specific IgE (sIgE) determination provides quantitative information. The main disadvantage of the available extract-based methods such as SPT is the variability of the crude extracts from different manufacturers available in the market, concordance limitations and cross-reactivity [7]. In children with persistent asthma, the characterisation of an atopic status is complex and often requires in vivo and in vitro tests [7,8].

There is still no consensus on the underlying pathophysiological basis of childhood asthma. Underlying chronic inflammation is often characterised by eosinophilic activity and allergic inflammation, but non-allergic asthma is not uncommon in childhood [9,10]. In addition, childhood asthma poses a significant clinical challenge in the diagnostic process, prognosis, and follow-up [10,11]. Inflammatory biomarker testing may provide additional information for the clinical evaluation and monitoring of children with asthma and respiratory allergies [7,12]. Therefore, at school age, the combined use of atopy biomarkers—sensitisation to allergens (SPT or serum sIgE), FeNO (fractional exhaled nitric oxide) and blood eosinophilia, can determine the risk of developing asthma in school-age and evaluate the severity of childhood asthma [2,12–14].

In children with asthma, the presence of atopy complicates achieving and maintaining good control [1,15]. On the other hand, allergic sensitization is a dynamic condition [16]. Additionally, monosensitized children may become polysensitized over time [16,17]. Therefore, experts recommend testing for inhalation and food allergens at least once per year (SPT and or serum sIgE), or more often in case of a new clinical allergic presentation [1,15]. The Monitoring asthma in children European Respiratory Society (ERS) Task Force recommends an active screening for allergen exposure, emerging sensitisation, or related changes in the clinical course of allergic disease [15]. The presence of allergies in patients with asthma (identified by SPT or serum sIgE) may help to identify the risk factors provoking asthma symptoms. A diagnostic clarification of atopy against particular food or aero-allergens is necessary, especially in the presence of suboptimal asthma control and before undertaking a change in therapy [1].

Historically, radioallergosorbent tests (RAST) have been the first to detect serum allergen-specific antibodies [6,18]. The first generation of quantitative tests (RAST, MAST—Multiple-antigen simultaneous test and EAST—Enzyme Allergosorbent Test) evolved into second-generation semi-quantitative IgE tests (AutoCAP, Alastat, HYTech, Matrix, MagicLite) to modern quality third-generation autoanalysers [6,19]. Two widely used third-generation immunological methods are the ImmunoCAP System (Phadia, Thermo Scientific, Uppsala, Sweden) and Immulite 2000 (Diagnostic Products Corporation, Los Angeles, CA, USA). The chemical analysis is similar to the original RAST, but non-isotopic markers are used; the study is faster, with improved precision, accuracy, and analytical sensitivity [20].

Multi-allergen screening tests are designed to measure sIgE against multiple allergens in a single assay. Allergens from different groups (house dust, animal epidermis, grass, tree pollen, fungal spores) or multiple allergens from the same group (e.g., mould—*Penicillium, Cladosporium, Alternaria, Aspergillus*) are embedded in a standard solid-phase [21]. Multi allergen screening for aero-allergens (Phadiatop), combined with a food allergen mix (fx5), is more effective than measuring individual allergen-specific IgE in characterising the atopic march of children with asthma [22]. These two tests showed a positive predictive value of 97.4% for any suspected allergic disease (asthma, AR, AD/eczema syndrome, food allergy) in children older than four [23,24]. Therefore, the combination of ImmunoCAP

Phadiatop (aeroallergens) with ImmunoCAP fx5 (food allergens) is officially accepted as the "gold standard" in clinical practice and in research determining the atopic status in childhood [25,26]. In addition, ImmunoCAP Phadiatop/fx5 has the highest predictive value for determining atopy from any available laboratory test (Phadiatop for children over 12 and in combination with fx5—under 12 years) [7,15].

2. Objectives

The study aims to perform a comparative analysis of the three laboratory methods for the serological assessment of the atopic status (the "gold standard" RAST multi-screening test ImmunoCAP Phadiatop/fx5, EAST Euroimmun pediatric immunoblot and total IgE ELISA) in children with bronchial asthma. Furthermore, we aimed to assess the clinical significance of atopic status determination in the enrolled children, based on serological testing (total serum IgE and sIgE) and history data for clinical manifestations of an allergy.

3. Materials and Methods

3.1. Subjects

In the study, 86 children with diagnosed bronchial asthma aged from 5 to 16 years were enrolled, in which 28 girls (33%) and 58 boys (67%), were hospitalised due to asthma exacerbation.

Before inclusion in the study and the collection of blood samples, all parents and children over 12 years of age signed a written Informed Consent, following the Commission on Ethics of Research at Medical University Sofia (Ethical approval No. 5/17.04.2013, scientific project identification code 23D/2013).

3.2. Study Design

All patients had a detailed medical history and were tested for total serum IgE antibodies by ELISA, EUROIMMUN Medizinische Labordiagnostica AG and specific IgE antibodies (Euroline Allergy Profile Pediatrics, Enzyme Allergo Sorbent Test (EAST) of Euroimmune® (Medizinische Labordiagnostica, AG, 2014, Luebeck, Germany). Additionally, the blood samples of 48 randomly selected children (18 girls and 30 boys with a mean age of 10.65 ± 4.14 SD) were assessed with a semi-quantitative in vitro assay of specific human IgE antibodies against a complex of food and aero-allergens in serum, by two different laboratory methods: Euroimmune® EUROLINE Pediatrics (Medizinische Labordiagnostica, AG, 2014, Luebeck, Germany) and Phadiatop/fx5 (multi-screening test for atopy) ImmunoCAP, Phadia, Thermo Fischer Scientific Inc., (Phadia AB®, Uppsala, Sweden) (Figure 1). The laboratory tests were performed by two independent certified laboratories in clinical immunology—Euroimmun Euroline Allergy Profile Pediatrics and total IgE in the Laboratory of Clinical Immunology of the University Hospital "St. Ivan Rilski" and ImmunoCAP Phadiatop/fx5 in the Laboratory of the Clinic of Clinical Immunology, University Hospital "Alexandrovska".

We defined the children as allergic and non-allergic according to the medical history data for diagnosed allergic disease, or clinically allergic manifestation prior to enrolment. Using an in vitro atopy diagnostic panel (serum total IgE and sIgE), we determined the children as atopic and non-atopic.

3.3. Laboratory Immunological Methods

o   Determination of serum levels of total IgE by ELISA (enzyme-linked immunosorbent assay), EUROIMMUN Medizinische Labordiagnostica AG

IgE concentration is determined using a calibration curve. The reading is performed at a 450/630 nm wavelength with four standards (calibrators) 0 U/mL, 10 U/mL, 100 U/mL, and 500 U/mL. Results are quantitative and are presented in U/mL. Normal values were determined relative to the upper limit of normal according to age. (Table S1).

o   Euroimmun EUROLINE Pediatric (complex of the most common food and aeroallergens in childhood).

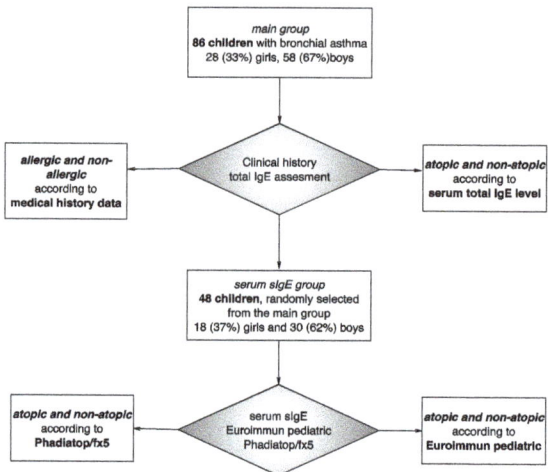

Figure 1. Study design.

EUROLINE test kits provided a semi-quantitative in vitro assay of human IgE antibodies in serum or plasma. It is a comprehensive screening profile with essential inhalation and food allergens for childhood allergies. The test strips are first activated with a universal buffer and then incubated at the first reaction with the patient's sera. If there are specific IgE antibodies in the test serum, they bind to the allergen. A second incubation is performed with enzyme-labeled monoclonal human IgE (enzyme conjugate) to visualise the bound antibodies, catalysing the enzymatic reaction. At the bottom of each test, there is a strip that acts as an indicator bar, representing the internal laboratory quality control. The colour reaction of the control indicator strip only becomes visible when the incubation is carried out correctly.

The EUROLINE test is a semi-quantitative method. The scale for reporting the results is expressed in the EAST system in seven classes—from 0 to 6 (<0.35 kU/L EAST class 0 to >100 kU/L EAST class6) (Table S2). Digital reporting of the results is performed with a scanning device (Canon®, Tokyo, Japan) and a licensed software product EUROLineScan program.

Allergens contained in the test membrane strips, include EUROLINE Pediatric (11 aero-allergens, 15 food allergen and CCD (cross-reactive carbohydrate determinants) marker) (Figure 2). Aero-allergens: gx grass mix 2 (timothy grass, cultivated rye), t3 birch, w6 mugwort, d1 *der. pteronyssinus*, d2 *der. farinae*, e1 cat, e2 dog, e3 horse, m2 *cladisporium her.*, m3 *aspergillus fum.*, m6 *alternaria* alt. Food allergens include f1 egg white, f75 egg yolk, f2 cow's milk, f3 codfish, f76 α-lactoalbumin, f77 β- lactoglobulin, f78 casein, e204 bovine serum albumin, f4 wheat flour, f9 rice, f14 soybean, f13 peanut, f17 hazelnut, f31 carrot, f35 potato, f49 apple, CCD marker, indicator band. CCDs can be found in various allergens from plant and animal origin. As a result of significant structural similarity, CCDs can cause strong cross-reactivity.

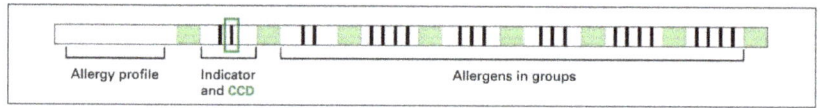

Figure 2. The principal structure of the membrane strip with allergen Euroimmun blot.

In order to perform a comparative analysis, we divided Euroimmun EUROLINE Pediatric into two groups—Euroimmun aero and Euroimmun food, depending on the inhaled and alimentary allergens.

o   Specific IgE—multi-screening atopy test—ImmunoCAP, Phadia (Thermo Fischer Scientific Inc, Phadia® AB, Uppsala, Sweden), Phadiatop (aeroallergen complex), and fx5 (MultiCAP food mix)

A Phadiatop test is a mixture of the following allergens: micro-mites (d), moulds (m), wood (t) and grass (g) allergens, weeds (w), animal allergens—dogs and cats (e). MultiCAP food mix (fx5) is the most commonly used pediatric multi-screening test for food allergy. It includes the following six food allergens—cow's milk protein, chicken egg white, white flour, fish, peanuts, and soy protein, which account for 90% of IgE-mediated food allergies in childhood.

The results of ImmunoCAP specific allergen mixtures are presented qualitatively (positive/negative/borderline) and quantitively (Specific IgE Class 0 to 6). Values between the lower limit of antibody detection and 0.35 kUA/l may indicate the presence of low IgE levels (class 1). Values $\geq$ 0.35 kUA/l indicate the occurrence of specific IgE antibodies against one or more allergens included in the multiallergen mixture. Healthy individuals have low levels of specific IgE in the peripheral blood, normally below 0.35 kUA/l (class 0). Sensitized patients show elevated levels, i.e., $\geq$0.35 kUA/l (class 1 to 6). The higher the value of the reported IgE kUA/l, the stronger the allergenic sensitisation (Table S3).

3.4. Statistical Methods

Raw data processing was performed with SPSS®, IBM 2009, version 19 (2010) and Excel (v. 2010). We used the methods of descriptive statistics to describe demographic and clinical characteristics of patients and the studied immunological parameters. We used a correlation analysis—between category characteristics (χ-square for more than two groups of one of the variables and Fisher's Exact test for tables with dimension 2 × 2); between categorical and quantitative features (Analysis of variance—ANOVA) and between quantitative features (correlation and regression analysis) to determine the existence of a relationship (associative or causal) between two or more indicators, its strength, shape and direction. When studying the specificity and sensitivity of quantitative diagnostic tests, we applied the method of ROC curves (Receiver operating characteristic), which represent the relationship between sensitivity (really positive values) as a function of 1-specificity (false positive values) Graphically.

4. Results

4.1. Demographic Characteristics

A total of 86 children were enrolled in the study and included in the main study group. All of them were diagnosed with bronchial asthma and hospitalised due to the exacerbation of symptoms. The children are 5 to 16 years old (mean age 10.18 (SD 3.54). Girls are 28 (33%) with a mean age of 9.98 (SD 3.41), and boys—58 (67%), mean age of 10.54 (SD 3.75).

Children aged 7 to 15 years predominate; 12.9% are pre-school age, and 8% are over 15 years old. Family history for bronchial asthma was reported in almost half of the children—48.8% (n 42), and 25.6% (n 22) of the children were in the first line relatives (mother, father, siblings). In 16 children, there was evidence of bronchial asthma in more than one family member. Approximately half of the children (48.8%) in the main group had medical history for allergy symptoms and/or a diagnosis prior the enrollment (AD, AR, food, drug, venom allergy, urticaria, angioedema). (Table 1) We defined these children as allergic. Concomitant AR was diagnosed in 46.4%.

Table 1. Children with atopic symptoms and or concomitant AR in the main study group.

According to the Medical History	Girls N 28	Boys N 58	Total N 86
Prior allergy symptoms	14 (50.0%)	28 (48.2%)	42 (48.8%)
Concomitant AR	13 (46.4%)	34 (58,6%)	47 (54.7%)

4.2. Total Serum IgE Determination (ELISA)

Serums of 86 children (main study group) were tested for total IgE level, 28 of whom were girls (33%) and 58 were boys (67%). Elevated IgE above the age-adjusted upper limit of normal was found in 64% ($n = 55$) of children: 67.8% ($n = 19$) girls and 62% ($n = 36$) boys. Very high levels of total IgE (titre ≥ 300 U/mL) were found in 35 children (40.1%).

The mean value of total IgE increases parallel with age in the studied group of asthmatic children, except for those older than 16 years, whose confidence interval was wide and uninformative (Figure 3). The mean value of total IgE in girls is slightly higher than that in boys, without significance ($p < 0.05$) (Table S4).

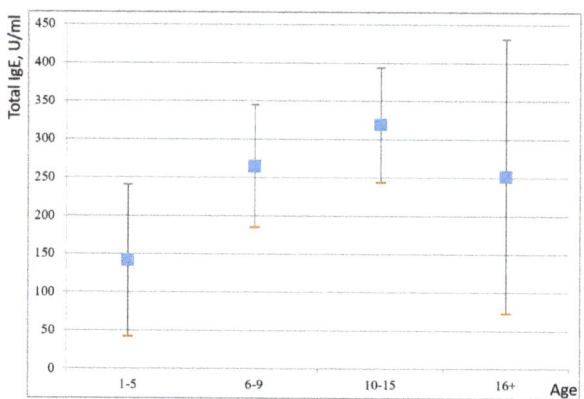

Figure 3. Serum level of total IgE.

- Comparative analysis of serum total IgE and sIgE, assessed by two methods (ImmunoCAP Phadiatop/fx5 and Euroimmun pediatric immunoblot)

In the serum sIgE group, 75 children (87%) showed elevated specific IgE (EUROIMMUN Pediatric). In addition, 27 children (32%) had normal total IgE antibodies (below age-related upper limit of normal—ULN) but at least one positive sIgE according the multiscreen (Phadiatop/fx5 and or Euroimmun pediatric). Of the children with elevated total IgE ($n = 55$), only 3 (5.5%) were negative for the studied sIgE panels (food and aeroallergens).

We constructed an ROC curve to determine the specificity and sensitivity of the serum level of total IgE in detecting children with atopy, defined as the positivity of specific IgE antibodies by both methods—EUROIMMUN Pediatric and ImmunoCAP Phadiatop/fx5. The ROC curve of total IgE against the multiscreen allergy test ImmunoCAP Phadiatop/fx5 ("gold standard") has an area under the curve of 0.667 (95% CI 0.500–0.834, $p = 0.073$, stand.err—0.085) (Figure 4a). The ROC curve of total IgE against the Euroimmun pediatrics (right) has an area under the curve (AUC) of 0.760 (95% CI 0.618–0.903, $p = 0.004$, stand.err—0.073) (Figure 4b).

At a threshold for total IgE above 368.5 U/mL, the method showed the best combination of sensitivity (50.5%) and specificity (81.8%), with 53.1 positive predictive value (PPV) and 86.6 negative predictive value (NPV) relative to the "gold standard" ImmunoCAP Phadiatop/fx5. However, even at a high titer of total IgE, the sensitivity remains relatively low (50.5%).

The ROC curve of total IgE compared to the Euroimmun paediatrics has better diagnostic characteristics, with a larger area under the AUC curve of 0.760 (95% CI 0.618–0.903). The threshold for total IgE over 142.5 combines best sensitivity (75%) and specificity (66.7%) in predicting the presence of positive specific IgE with 83.2 PPV of 51.7.

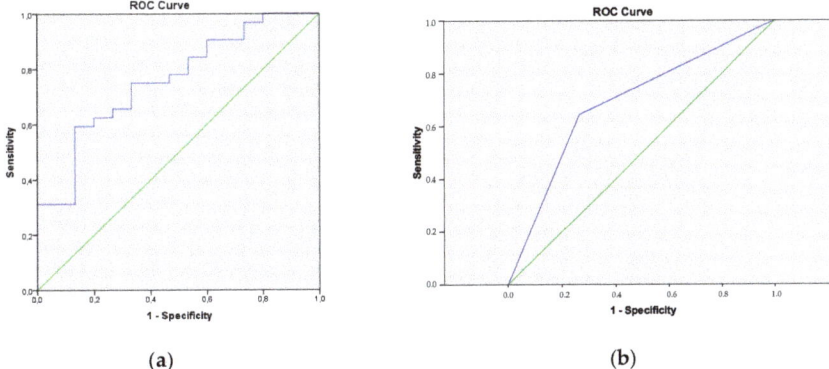

Figure 4. ROC curve to assess the specificity and sensitivity of total IgE vs. ImmunoCAP Phadiatop/fx5 (**a**) and total IgE vs. Euroimmun paediatrics (**b**).

The elevated specific IgE against *D. pteronyssimus* ($p < 0.0001$), *D. farinae* ($p < 0.0001$) for titers above 1 EAST class, and against cat fur with titers above 3 EAST class, correlate with the level of total IgE ($p = 0.009$) (Table S5).

- Comparative analysis of serum sIgE against aero-allergens, assessed by two methods (ImmunoCAP Phadiatop and Euroimmun aero)

We constructed an ROC curve to determine the sensitivity and specificity of EUROIMMUN aero to ImmunoCAP Phadiatop (the 'gold standard') (Figure 5). The ROC curve shows AUC—0.958 (Stand.error—0.026, 95% CI (0.000–1.000), $p = 0.000$).

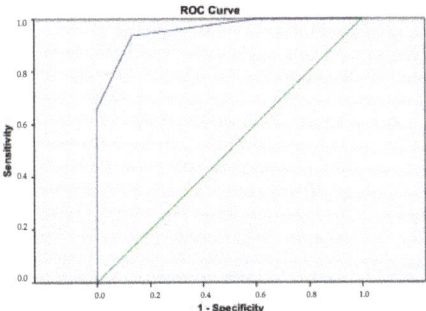

Figure 5. ROC curve for assessing the specificity and sensitivity of Euroimmun aero (as a panel positive/negative) vs. ImmunoCAP Phadiatop.

In multiple analyses for single aero-allergens included in EUROIMMUN aero, the ROC curves remain significant. Aero-allergens d2, e1 and gx are characterised by low sensitivity (between 40 and 60%) and high specificity (above 80%) at EAST class 1 (Figure 6 and Table S6a,b).

Other aero-allergens included in EUROIMMUN aero (dog, birch, and wild wormwood) did not show good predictive value with an area under the curve of below 0.5 (Table S6a,b).

There was a moderate to strong correlation between sIgE titer (e1, d1, d2 and gx) assessed by ImmunoCAP Phadiatop and Euroimmun aero. (Table S7).

- Comparative analysis of specific IgE against food allergens, assessed by two methods (ImmunoCAP fx5 and Euroimmun food)

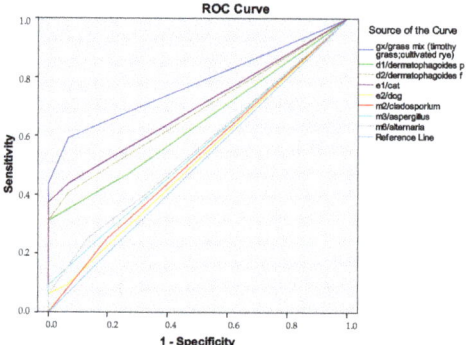

Figure 6. ROC curve for assessing the specificity and sensitivity of EUROIMMUN aero (distinct sIgE) vs. ImmunoCAP Phadiatop.

There was a moderate to strong correlation between the sIgE titer determined with ImmunoCap fx5 (food mix) and those with Euroimmun food—soy (soybean), flour ($p = 0.006$), rice ($p = 0.090$), apple ($p = 0.007$), as well as a weak correlation for peanut. However, no statistically significant correlation was found between the two methods for other food allergens included in the fx5 mix (Table S8).

We constructed an ROC curve to determine the sensitivity and specificity of EUROIMMUN food to ImmunoCAP fx5. Values of EUROIMMUN food above 1 EAST class have a sensitivity of 64.3% and a 73.5% specificity with AUC—0.689, stand. error—0.087, 95% CI (0.518–0.860), $p = 0.041$ (Figure 7a). To check which IgE to use from the EUROIMMUN food to predict the ImmunoCAP fx5 positivity, we performed a multiple analysis with an ROC curve (Figure 7b) and (Table S9).

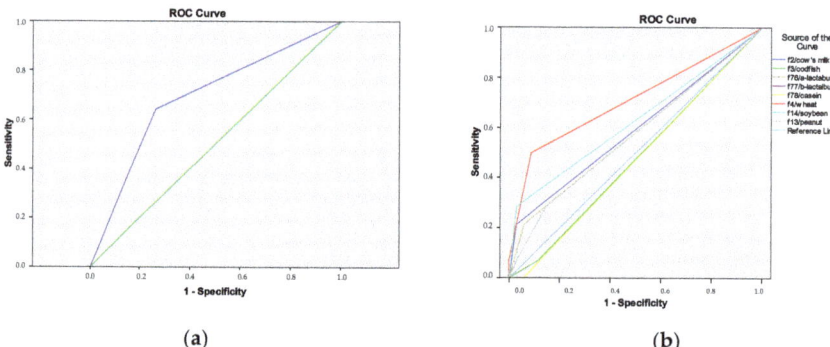

(a) (b)

Figure 7. ROC curve for assessment of the specificity and sensitivity of EUROIMMUN food (as a panel positive/negative) to ImmunoCAP fx5 (**a**), ROC curve for evaluation of the specificity and sensitivity of EUROIMMUN food (distinct sIgE) to ImmunoCAP fx5 (**b**).

When combining milk allergens (f2, f76, f77, f 78) in one variable, the predictive value increases (Table 2).

Table 2. Characteristics of the ROC curve—multiple analysis, cow milk as a combined variable.

Tested Allergen	AUC	SE		95% CI	
				Lower Limit	Upper Limit
f2,f76,f77,f78	0.620	0.095	0.196	0.434	0.805

- Clinical significance of medical history, total IgE and sIgE, assessed by two methods

No significant difference was found between mean titer level of total IgE and Phadiatop/fx5 in children with and without a family history of atopy ($p > 0.05$). For total IgE, the difference is borderline but not significant ($p = 0.077$). In addition, no significant difference was found in mean serum levels of total IgE in the groups of children with and without history data for a clinically manifested allergy (allergic children) ($p > 0.05$).

In the studied population of children, the family history for asthma was associated with clinical symptoms of allergic diseases (AD, drug and food allergies). ($p = 0.048$) Additionally, family history for atopy shows a tendency to correlate with positivity for sIgE antibodies against cat. ($p = 0.054$).

There was a significant difference in total IgE levels in children with and without AR, but not in groups with and without other allergic symptoms/diseases. The mean value of total IgE is significantly higher in children with asthma and AR than in those without concomitant AR. (mean 202.52, IQR 102.50 (24.20–363.95) vs. 316.68, IQR 261.00 (109.20–552.50) ($p = 0.005$).

There was a significant difference in mean serum levels of total IgE in the group of atopic and non-atopic children according to Euroimmun paediatrics sIgE. Atopic children have a significantly higher total IgE titer than non-atopic children (mean 52.4, IQR 39.50 (8.50–83.40) vs. mean 293 IQR (261.00 (91.30–549.60) ($p < 0.0001$).

The chi-square analysis showed that among the group of polysensitised (more than 2 positive sIgE) children, more patients with high or borderline IgE were observed than non-atopic or monosensitised patients (at least one positive sIgE) ($p = 0.003$) (Figure S1).

Overall, 70% (N 14) of children who were defined as allergic according to the medical history had a positive Phadiatop/fx5 result, and 35.7% of the non-allergic according to their history had a negative test result.

Phadiatop/fx5 identified 36 children as atopic and 16 as non-atopic. In 9 children (56%) identified as non-atopic with Phadiatop/fx5, at least one positive sIgE antibody was detected with EUROIMMUN Pediatric (7 of them with EAST class 1, only two with EAST class 2). On the other hand, two children (5.6%) identified as atopic with Phadiatop/fx5 showed a negative result with the EUROIMMUN Pediatric. (only food allergens EAST class 1).

Medical history for allergy symptoms (drug, food, venom allergy, urticaria, AD, angioedema) were reported in 20 children (41%). In two (10%) of the children, atopy was not confirmed with EUROIMMUN Pediatric and ImmunoCAP. The total IgE was increased in 52% ($n = 25$) of children and defined the children as atopic. Using the Phadiatop/fx5, 75% of the tested children ($n = 36$) were classified as atopic, and 85.4% ($n = 41$) with EUROIMMUN Pediatric.

In the serum sIgE group, 28 (58.3%) children had concomitant AR. According to medical history, 46%, are allergic according to the total IgE titer—71% are atopic, Phadiatop/fx5—86%, and EUROIMMUN Pediatric—92.8% (Figure S2).

5. Discussion

Serological diagnosis of atopy began in 1968, and demonstrated a link between the body's sensitisation and the newly discovered class of human immunoglobulins called IgE [27]. Serum concentrations of total IgE are known to have high specificity but low sensitivity in determining atopic status. Thus, in the presence of elevated total IgE, the patient is likely to be atopic, but if normal, atopy cannot be ruled out [12,15]. This was supported by our results. Both analyses of ROC curves, using the two methods for detecting sIgE as a reference, showed excellent specificity but low sensitivity even at high titers for total IgE (>142.5 U/mL and >368.5 U/mL, respectively).

Total IgE levels among atopic children correlate with the size of the target organ, with the lowest values reported in individuals with AR, the highest in those with AD and intermediate for asthmatics [27]. According to our results, the total IgE value is significantly higher in children with asthma and AR than in those without concomitant AR. ($p = 0.005$). Using an χ square, we observed more patients with high or borderline IgE in the group of polysensitised children than in the non-atopic or monosensitised. ($p = 0.003$).

In healthy subjects, total IgE levels increase from birth (0–1 KU/l) to adolescence, decreasing slowly until reaching a plateau at 20–30 years [6,18,28]. Our results confirmed a significant increase in total IgE mean value with age, except for those over 16 years, whose confidence interval is uninformatively wide [6].

In order to define the allergen avoiding strategy, international guidelines include sIgE assessments to identify the subject's comorbidity [29,30]. However, literature data indicate that multi-allergens screening methods detecting aeroallergen in combination with a food allergen mix are more effective than measuring individual allergen-specific IgE in characterising the atopic status of children with asthma [7].

Allergen-specific IgE have a significant advantage, especially in detecting children with clinically undiagnosed allergies. In the studies population, 73% of hildren had positive sIgE. However, only half of them have a positive history of allergies. Furthermore, a higher percentage of children are sensitised to aero-allergens (64%) than those sensitised against food allergens (43%). This ratio corresponds to literature data for the tested age group. In contrast, atopic sensitisation for food allergens predominates in infants [31,32].

In a recently published study, Chang et al. investigated the sensitivity and specificity of Phadiatop and total IgE levels in hospitalised adults and children with clinical symptoms, suggesting persistent allergic rhinitis. In the study, 576 children were enrolled. The authors report sensitivities and specificities of 86.3% and 77.4% of the total IgE levels to predict positive allergens using Phadiatop in children, and 65.7% and 85.7%, respectively, in adults [33]. Pierotti et al. performed a cross-sectional study of Brazilian children, who were tested for total IgE using Phadiatop and Phadiatop infant. They found a significantly higher mean total serum level of IgE among allergic children, especially those with asthma/rhinitis, as confirmed by our results [34]. Khasawaneh et al. estimated the sensitivity and specificity of total IgE as 77.4% and 92.5%, respectively, when using sIgE as a standard test. The authors tested 80 patients between 1 year and 77 years, 32 of whom were children. Specific IgE were tested with immunoblot EUROLINE. Our result has shown lower sensitivity (50.5%) and similar specificity (81.8%) of the total IgE (the threshold for total IgE above 368.5 U/mL) to predict a positive ImmunoCap Phadiatop result. We found better sensitivity (75%) and lower specificity (66.%) in the total IgE as a predictor for positive Euroimmun paediatrics, using 142.5 U/mL as an LLN for the IgE total (larger area under the AUC curve of 0.760) [23].

When compared the sensitivity and specificity of EUROIMMUN aero vs. the "gold standard" ImmunoCAP Phadiatop, we found 100% sensitivity, but only 40% specificity (PPV 68.1%, NPV 100%) for EUROIMMUN aero using EAST class 1 as a tress hold and 98.3% sensitivity and 87, 6% specificity (PPV 94.4%, NPV 96%) for values greater than EAST class 2, which is similar to the results reported in the literature [23,25]. ROC curves remain significant only for *D. Farinae*, cat, and grass mix in multiple aero-allergens analyses. For all other aero-allergens included in the panel (dog, birch, and wild wormwood), EUROIMMUN aero did not show good predictive properties. According to the manufacturer data, the sensitivity of EUROLINE to the Phadia CAP system („gold standard") for timothy (grass) and birch is 90%, for *D. Pteronyssimus* and *D. Farinae* it is 83% and 84%, respectively, for cat it is 91% and for horse it is 100%. Thus, the two methods have similar indicators in terms of general sensitivity and specificity [35].

Compared to ImmunoCAP fx5 food mix (cow's milk protein, wheat, chicken egg white, fish, peanuts, and soybeans), EUROIMMUN food showed weaker but acceptable sensitivity at 64.3% and specificity of 73.5%, including for lower titers (EAST class 1). In the multiple analysis, the highest predictive power had an sIgE against flour and soy and them combined, but a single sIgE against allergens in cow's milk (f2, f76, f77, f78).

The presence of positive sIgE using the Euroimmun aero was detected in 9 children, which result was negative when using the ImmunoCAP Phadiatop. Seven of them had a sIgE titer corresponding to Euroimmun immunoblot EAST class 1 and only two to EAST class 2. The main sIgE positive with both methods are from the mould group—*Cladosporium* and *Alternaria*. According to data from patient history, 41.7% of the children are atopic (with clinically manifested allergy).

Total IgE levels showed an increased age-related serum titer in 52% of the tested children, and serological tests for sIgE determined an additional 23 to 30% of children as atopic. According to the Phadiatop/fx5 result, 75% of the children are atopic, using EUROIMMUN Pediatric the percentage of atopic children was found to be 85.4%. In children with concomitant AR, the detectability of atopy by serological methods in children without a history of allergies is even more significant. Singh et al. found Phadiatop/fx5 to reveal that physicians' diagnosis of IgE mediated allergy is accurate in only 59% of cases in the Indian study of allergen sensitisation prevalence. We found that the case history alone reveals atopic children with asthma and concomitant AR in 46% and even in lower per cent 41.7 in the group of asthmatic children without AR [36]. According to data cited by the manufacturer, ImmunoCAP Phadiatop demonstrated 91% specificity, 89% efficacy, and 91% correct classification of patients (atopic/non-atopic) in a study of 836 patients with allergy-related symptoms in six different centres (Italy, Spain, Germany, the Netherlands, Sweden, Great Britain) [20,37]. The study used a threshold for the specific IgE calibrator with a value of 0.35 kUA/l, used in the present study [30].

The results of our study showed an excellent correlation between the two serological methods in terms of sensitivity and specificity. EUROIMMUN Pediatric demonstrated an advantage over the "gold standard" in detecting children with atopy. Using correlation, regression, and factor analyses, we found that ImmunoCAP Phadiatop/fx5 missed positive results in 19% of patients compared to the EUROIMMUN Pediatric results. This error is weaker for fx5 than Phadiatop, probably due to the broader aero-allergenic spectrum embedded in the EUROIMMUN panel. ImmunoCAP Phadiatop and fx5 generate a dichotomous positive/negative value and relative positivity semi-quantitatively (kilo units per litre). Thus the summary result does not define which of the included sIgE is positive. On the other hand, EUROIMMUN Pediatric offers a broader range of tested allergens—inhaled and food allergens with comparable sensitivity and the ability to detect the specific allergen(s) responsible for the positive result. Additionally, EUROIMMUN Pediatric provides a titer for each particular sIgE (semi-quantitative, expressed in EAST class system), not a summary result as provided by ImmunoCAP Phadiatop/fx5.

Skevaki et al. compared the three commonly used technologies for sIgE detection—ImmunoCAP™ sx1 and fx5 mixes, the ImmunoCAP ISAC™ 112 microarray and a Euroline™ panel. Euroline identified the highest percentage of positive samples out of 12 comparable allergens. However, the authors found that, when considering the overall positive samples, Euroline suffers from a higher background signal. In addition, it detects the highest number of sensitisations at threshold 1, but not at a higher and more stringent threshold [38].

Another advantage of EUROIMMUN pediatric immunoblot is the user-friendly and straightforward methodology, which does not require specialised and expensive equipment, easily applicable in daily clinical and laboratory practice. Combined with the excellent specificity and sensitivity of the method and the reliability of results, it is a reasonable alternative to the ImmunoCAP methods. Additionally, we confirmed the correlation between elevated total IgE and the history data for symptoms suggestive of allergic disease. However, total IgE titer is significantly less sensitive than serological multiscreen atopy tests (sIgE panels).

6. Limitation of the Study

We must acknowledge that the results are based on a small number of patients positive for specific IgE against food allergens, which may affect the objectivity of the analysis. Additionally, significant titers (>3.5 IU/mL) were detected only for aero-allergens by both methods (ImmunoCAP, EUROIMMUN). In addition, sIgE detected against food allergens had low titers—EAST class 1 and 2, less than 3.5 kUA/L; kU/L). Lastly, we included children with asthma with/without AR, but we did not have healthy controls. Therefore, we believe that the study's limitations do not make it invalid, but they are opportunities to inspire future research.

7. Conclusions

Contact with provocative allergen(s) in sensitised children with bronchial asthma and respiratory allergy is a risk factor for exacerbation/hospitalisation. Allergen-specific IgEs have a significant advantage, especially in the detection of children with clinically undiagnosed allergies. Identifying sIgE for particular allergens is essential for the effective management of asthma and other allergic diseases—prevention, diagnosis, and treatment. EUROIMMUN blot methodology does not require specialised equipment and is easily applicable in everyday clinical and laboratory practice. Combined with its high reliability, it makes it an affordable alternative to the "gold standard" ImmunoCAP.

Supplementary Materials: The following are available online at https://www.mdpi.com/article/10.3390/sinusitis6010001/s1, Table S1: Reference values for specific IgE in serum, Table S2: EAST scale for reporting the results, Table S3: ImmunoCAP reading scale (kUA/l) * The expected values for specific IgE are not age-dependent, Table S4: Comparison of mean total IgE (U/ml) titer values by sex (girls/boys), Table S5: Comparison of the mean values of total IgE between positive specific IgE against cats and house dust mites against children with a negative test, Table S6: a. ROC curve characteristics of EUROIMMUN aero vs ImmunoCAP Phadiatop, b. ROC curve characteristics of EUROIMMUN aero vs. ImmunoCAP Phadiatop, Table S7: Correlation analysis between ImmunoCAP Phadiatop and Euroimmun aero, Table S8: Correlation analysis between ImmunoCAP Phadiatop and Euroimmun food, Table S9: ROC curve characteristics (assessment of the specificity and sensitivity of EUROIMMUN food to ImmunoCAP fx5), Figure S1. Comparison of total IgE titer in the group of non-atopic, mono- and polysensitised patients, Euroimmun pediatrics, $p = 0.003$, Figure S2. Classification of children with bronchial asthma and AR as atopic / non-atopic (N = 28).

Author Contributions: Conceptualisation, S.L. and T.V.; Data curation, M.B. and E.N.; Formal analysis, S.L., M.B., S.P. and E.N.; Funding acquisition, S.L.; Investigation, S.L. and T.V.; Methodology, S.L., M.B. and T.V.; Project administration, S.L.; Resources, T.V.; Software, S.P. and E.N.; Supervision, T.V.; Validation, S.L. and E.N.; Visualization, S.P. and T.V.; Writing—original draft, S.L. and T.V.; Writing—review and editing, S.L., S.P. and T.V. All authors have read and agreed to the published version of the manuscript.

Funding: This research was funded by a grant from the Medical University of Sofia (Council of Medical Science, project no. 35D/2013, grant no. 23D/2013).

Institutional Review Board Statement: The study was conducted according to the guidelines of the Declaration of Helsinki and approved by the Ethics Committee on Scientific Research at Medical University of Sofia (ethical approval No. 5/17.04.2013, scientific project identification code 23D/2013).

Informed Consent Statement: Before the study enrolment, all parents and children over 12 years old signed written informed consent and child assent, according to the Ethics Committee on Scientific Research requirements at the Medical University of Sofia.

Data Availability Statement: Data available on request due to restrictions, e.g., privacy or ethics.

Acknowledgments: We want to thank Diana Hristova, clinical allergologist for the help in the review process.

Conflicts of Interest: The authors declare no conflict of interest.

References

1. Pijnenburg, M.W.; Baraldi, E.; Brand, P.L.; Carlsen, K.-H.; Eber, E.; Frischer, T.; Hedlin, G.; Kulkarni, N.; Lex, C.; Mäkelä, M.J.; et al. Monitoring Asthma in Children. *Eur. Respir. J.* **2015**, *25*, 178–186. [CrossRef] [PubMed]
2. Nelson, H.S.; Szefler, S.J.; Jacobs, J.; Huss, K.; Shapiro, G.; Sternberg, A.L. The relationships among environmental allergen sensitization, allergen exposure, pulmonary function, and bronchial hyperresponsiveness in the Childhood Asthma Management Program. *J. Allergy Clin. Immunol.* **1999**, *104*, 775–785. [CrossRef]
3. Justiz Vaillant, A.A.; Modi, P.; Jan, A. *StatPearls*; StatPearls Publishing: Treasure Island, FL, USA, 2021. Available online: https://www.ncbi.nlm.nih.gov/books/NBK542187/ (accessed on 20 December 2021).

4. Thomsen, S.F. Epidemiology and natural history of atopic diseases. *Eur. Clin. Respir. J.* **2015**, *2*, 24642. [CrossRef]
5. Ahmed, H.; Ospina, M.B.; Sideri, K.; Vliagoftis, H. Retrospective analysis of aeroallergen's sensitization patterns in Edmonton, Canada. *Allergy Asthma Clin. Immunol.* **2019**, *15*, 6. [CrossRef]
6. Ansotegui, I.J.; Melioli, G.; Canonica, G.W.; Caraballo, L.; Villa, E.; Ebisawa, M.; Passalacqua, G.; Savi, E.; Ebo, D.; Gómez, R.M.; et al. IgE allergy diagnostics and other relevant tests in allergy, a World Allergy Organization position paper. *World Allergy Organ. J.* **2020**, *13*, 100080, Erratum in **2021**, *14*, 100557. [CrossRef]
7. Szefler, S.J.; Wenzel, S.; Brown, R.; Erzurum, S.C.; Fahy, J.V.; Hamilton, R.G.; Hunt, J.F.; Kita, H.; Liu, A.H.; Panettieri, R.A.; et al. Asthma outcomes: Biomarkers. *J. Allergy Clin. Immunol.* **2012**, *129*, S9–S23. [CrossRef] [PubMed]
8. Sly, P.; Boner, A.L.; Björksten, B.; Bush, A.; Custovic, A.; Eigenmann, P.; Gern, J.E.; Gerritsen, J.; Hamelmann, E.; Helms, P.J.; et al. Early identification of atopy in the prediction of persistent asthma in children. *Lancet* **2008**, *372*, 1100–1106. [CrossRef]
9. Garcia, G.V.; Blake, K. Considerations for the Child with Nonatopic Asthma. *Pediatr. Allergy Immunol. Pulmonol.* **2020**, *33*, 39–42. [CrossRef] [PubMed]
10. Holguin, F. The atopic march: IgE is not the only road. *Lancet Respir. Med.* **2014**, *2*, 88–90. [CrossRef]
11. Sinisgalli, S.; Collins, M.S.; Schramm, C.M. Clinical Features Cannot Distinguish Allergic from Non-allergic Asthma in Children. *J. Asthma* **2011**, *49*, 51–56. [CrossRef] [PubMed]
12. Sánchez-García, S.; Habernau Mena, A.; Quirce, S. Biomarkers in inflammometry pediatric asthma: Utility in daily clinical practice. *Eur. Clin. Respir. J.* **2017**, *4*, 1356160. [CrossRef] [PubMed]
13. Chang, D.; Yao, W.; Tiller, C.J.; Kisling, J.; Slaven, J.E.; Yu, Z.; Kaplan, M.H.; Tepper, R.S. Exhaled nitric oxide during infancy as a risk factor for asthma and airway hyperreactivity. *Eur. Respir. J.* **2015**, *45*, 98–106. [CrossRef]
14. Rø, A.D.; Simpson, M.R.; Storrø, O.; Johnsen, R.; Videm, V.; Øien, T. The predictive value of allergen skin prick tests and IgE tests at pre-school age: The PACT study. *Pediatr. Allergy Immunol.* **2014**, *25*, 691–698. [CrossRef] [PubMed]
15. Moeller, A.; Carlsen, K.H.; Sly, P.D.; Baraldi, E.; Piacentini, G.; Pavord, I.; Lex, C.; Saglani, S.; ERS Task Force Monitoring Asthma in Children. Monitoring asthma in childhood: Lung function, bronchial responsiveness and inflammation. *Eur. Respir. Rev.* **2015**, *136*, 204–215. [CrossRef]
16. Fasce, L.; Tosca, M.A.; Olcese, R.; Ciprandi, G.; Baroffio, M. Atopy in wheezing infants always starts with monosensitization. *Allergy Asthma Proc.* **2007**, *28*, 449–453. [CrossRef] [PubMed]
17. Migueres, M.; Dávila, I.; Frati, F.; Azpeitia, Y.; Jeanpetit, Y.; Lhéritier-Barrand, M.; Incorvaia, C.; Ciprandi, G.; PlurAL Study Group. Types of sensitization to aeroallergens: Definitions, prevalences and impact on the diagnosis and treatment of allergic respiratory disease. *Clin. Transl. Allergy* **2014**, *4*, 16. [CrossRef]
18. Burrows, B.; Martinez, F.D.; Cline, M.G.; Lebowitz, M.D. The relationship between parental and children's serum IgE and asthma. *Am. J. Respir. Crit. Care Med.* **1995**, *152*, 1497–1500. [CrossRef]
19. Hamilton, R.G. Microarray Technology Applied to Human Allergic Disease. *Microarrays* **2017**, *6*, 3. [CrossRef] [PubMed]
20. Paganelli, R.; Ansotegui, I.J.; Sastre, J.; Lange, C.-E.; Roovers, M.H.W.M.; de Groot, H.; Lindholm, N.B.; Ewan, P.W. Specific IgE antibodies in the diagnosis of atopic disease: Clinical evaluation of a new in vitro test system, UniCAP™, in six European allergy clinics. *Allergy* **2008**, *53*, 763–768. [CrossRef]
21. Wever, A.M.J.; Wever-Hess, J.; Van Schayck, C.P.; Van Weel, C. Evaluation of the Phadiatop® test in an epidemiological study. *Allergy* **1990**, *45*, 92–97. [CrossRef]
22. Liu, Y.-H.; Chou, H.-H.; Jan, R.-L.; Lin, H.-J.; Liang, C.-C.; Wang, J.-Y.; Wu, Y.-C.; Shieh, C.-C. Comparison of two specific allergen screening tests in different patient groups. *Acta Paediatr. Taiwan* **2006**, *47*, 116–122.
23. Khasawneh, R.; Hiary, M.; Abadi, B.; Salameh, A.; Moman, S. Total and Specific Immunoglobulin E for Detection of Most Prevalent Aeroallergens in a Jordanian Cohort. *Med. Arch.* **2019**, *73*, 272–275. [CrossRef]
24. Wickman, M.; Ahlstedt, S.; Lilja, G.; Hamsten, M.V.H. Quantification of IgE antibodies simplifies the classification of allergic diseases in 4-year-old children. A report from the prospective birth cohort study—BAMSE. *Pediatr. Allergy Immunol.* **2003**, *14*, 441–447. [CrossRef] [PubMed]
25. Zeng, G.; Hu, H.; Zheng, P.; Wu, G.; Wei, N.; Liang, X.; Sun, B.; Zhang, X. The practical benefit of Phadiatop test as the first-line in vitro allergen-specific immunoglobulin E (sIgE) screening of aeroallergens among Chinese asthmatics: A validation study. *Ann. Transl. Med.* **2018**, *6*, 151. [CrossRef] [PubMed]
26. Park, K.H.; Lee, J.; Sim, D.W.; Lee, S.C. Comparison of Singleplex Specific IgE Detection Immunoassays: ImmunoCAP Phadia 250 and Immulite 2000 3gAllergy. *Ann. Lab. Med.* **2018**, *38*, 23–31. [CrossRef]
27. Baldacci, S.; Omenaas, E.; Oryszczyn, M. Allergy markers in respiratory epidemiology. *Eur. Respir. J.* **2001**, *17*, 773–790. [CrossRef]
28. Hamilton, R.G.; Adkinson, N.F. In vitro assays for the diagnosis of IgE-mediated disorders. *J. Allergy Clin. Immunol.* **2004**, *114*, 213–225. [CrossRef]
29. Frith, J.; Fleming, L.; Bossley, C.; Ullmann, N.; Bush, A. The complexities of defining atopy in severe childhood asthma. *Clin. Exp. Allergy* **2011**, *41*, 948–953. [CrossRef]
30. Hamilton, R.G.; Matsson, P.N.; Hovanec-Burns, D.L.; Van Cleve, M.; Chan, S.; Kober, A.; Kleine-Tebbe, J.R.; Renz, H.; Magnusson, C.; Quicho, R.; et al. Analytical Performance Characteristics, Quality Assurance and Clinical Utility of Immunological Assays for Human IgE Antibodies of Defined Allergen Specificities. (CLSI-ILA20-A3). *J. Allergy Clin. Immunol.* **2015**, *135*, AB8. [CrossRef]
31. Ferraro, V.; Zanconato, S.; Carraro, S. Timing of Food Introduction and the Risk of Food Allergy. *Nutrients* **2019**, *11*, 1131. [CrossRef]

32. Dhami, S.; Sheikh, A. Estimating the prevalence of aero-allergy and/or food allergy in infants, children and young people with moderate-to-severe atopic eczema/dermatitis in primary care: Multi-centre, cross-sectional study. *J. R. Soc. Med.* **2015**, *108*, 229–236. [CrossRef]
33. Chang, Y.-C.; Lee, T.-J.; Huang, C.-C.; Chang, P.-H.; Chen, Y.-W.; Fu, C.-H. The Role of Phadiatop Tests and Total Immunoglobulin E Levels in Screening Aeroallergens: A Hospital-Based Cohort Study. *J. Asthma Allergy* **2021**, *14*, 135–140. [CrossRef]
34. Pierotti, F.F.; Aranda, C.S.; Cocco, R.R.; Sarinho, E.; Sano, F.; Porto, A.; Rosário, N.; Neto, H.J.C.; Goudouris, E.; Moraes, L.S.; et al. Phadiatop, Phadiatop Infant and total IgE evaluated in allergic Brazilian children and adolescents. *Allergol. Immunopathol.* **2020**, *48*, 259–264. [CrossRef]
35. EUROLINE Pediatric (IgE) Test Instruction. Available online: http://shop.tinyteria.com/index.php?route=extension/module/free_downloads/download&did=1419 (accessed on 20 December 2021).
36. Singh, S. Asthma diagnosis and treatment—1001. Identification of prevalent sensitizing allergens in India. *World Allergy Organ. J.* **2013**, *6*, P1. [CrossRef]
37. Thermo. Available online: https://www.thermofisher.com/phadia/wo/en/our-solutions/immunocap-allergy-solutions/specific-ige-single-allergens/atopy.html (accessed on 20 December 2021).
38. Skevaki, C.; Tafo, P.; Eiringhaus, K.; Timmesfeld, N.; Weckmann, M.; Happle, C.; Nelson, P.P.; Maison, N.; Schaub, B.; Ricklefs, I.; et al. Allergen extract- and component-based diagnostics in children of the ALLIANCE asthma cohort. *Clin. Exp. Allergy* **2021**, *51*, 1331–1345. [CrossRef]

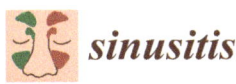 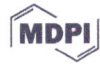

Article

Study of Nasal Fractional Exhaled Nitric Oxide (FENO) in Children with Allergic Rhinitis

Sy Duong-Quy [1,2,3,*,†], Thuy Nguyen-Thi-Dieu [4,†], Khai Tran-Quang [5], Tram Tang-Thi-Thao [1], Toi Nguyen-Van [1], Thu Vo-Pham-Minh [5], Quan Vu-Tran-Thien [6], Khue Bui-Diem [6], Vinh Nguyen-Nhu [6], Lam Hoang-Thi [7] and Timothy Craig [3]

1. Clinical Research Unit, Lam Dong Medical College and Bio-Medical Research Center, Dalat 84263, Vietnam; thaotram1989@gmail.com (T.T.-T.-T.); nguyentoi08@yahoo.com (T.N.-V.)
2. Internal Medicine Department, Pham Ngoc Thach Medical University, Ho Chi Minh City 8428, Vietnam
3. Immuno-Allergology Department, Hershey Medical Center, Penn State Medical College, State College, PA 16801, USA; tcraig@pennstatehealth.psu.edu
4. Department of Paediatrics, Hanoi Medical University, Hanoi 8424, Vietnam; nguyendieuthuyhmu@gmail.com
5. Internal medicine Department, Can Tho University of Medicine and Pharmacy, Can Tho 8492, Vietnam; tqkhai@ctump.edu.vn (K.T.-Q.); vpminhthu76@yahoo.com (T.V.-P.-M.)
6. Department of Lung Functional Testing, University of Medicine and Pharmacy, Ho Chi Minh City 8428, Vietnam; vutranthienquan@gmail.com (Q.V.-T.-T.); bui.diemkhue@gmail.com (K.B.-D.); vinhnguyenmd@ump.edu.vn (V.N.-N.)
7. Department of Immuno-Allergology, Hanoi Medical University, Hanoi 8424, Vietnam; bshoangthilam@gmail.com

* Correspondence: sduongquy.jfvp@gmail.com; Tel.: +84-918413813
† Co-first author.

Abstract: (1) Background: Exhaled nitric oxide (NO) has been considered as a biomarker of airway inflammation. The measurement of fractional exhaled NO (FENO) is a valuable test for assessing local inflammation in subjects with allergic rhinitis (AR). (2) Objective: To evaluate (a) the correlation between nasal FENO with anthropometric characteristics, symptoms of AR and nasal peak flows in children without and with AR; and (b) the cut-off of nasal FENO for diagnosis of AR in symptomatic children. (3) Methods: The study was a descriptive and cross-sectional study in subjects with and without AR < 18 years old. All clinical and functional characteristics of the study subjects were recorded for analysis. They were divided into healthy subjects for the control group and subjects with AR who met all inclusion criteria. (4) Results: 100 subjects (14 ± 3 years) were included, including 32 control subjects and 68 patients with AR. Nasal FENO in AR patients was significantly higher than in control subjects: 985 ± 232 ppb vs. 229 ± 65 ppb ($p < 0.001$). In control subjects, nasal FENO was not correlated with anthropometric characteristics and nasal inspiratory or expiratory peak flows (IPF or EPF) ($p > 0.05$). There was a correlation between nasal FENO and AR symptoms in AR patients and nasal IPF and EPF ($p = 0.001$ and 0.0001, respectively). The cut-off of nasal FENO for positive AR diagnosis with the highest specificity and sensitivity was ≥794 ppb (96.7% and 92.6%, respectively). (5) Conclusion: The use of nasal FENO as a biomarker of AR provides a useful tool and additional armamentarium in the management of allergic rhinitis.

Keywords: nitric oxide; NO; exhaled NO; FENO; allergic rhinitis; nasal peak flow

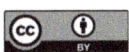

1. Introduction

In the upper airway, exhaled nitric oxide (NO) is produced mainly from the rhinosinusitis mucosa. It can be measured by non-invasive techniques using devices with chemiluminescence or electroluminescence methods [1–3]. The main source of nasal NO is consistently generated from the nasal mucosa and perinasal sinus epithelium, where inducible nitric oxide synthase (iNOS) is present. In the upper airway, the role of nasal NO has been described as regulating airway function, providing non-specific protection against infection related to its destructive property. Nasal NO also contributes to upper airway protection due to its role in regulating ciliary motility, and low nasal NO levels are usually associated with decreased upper airway ciliary function [4]. Nasal NO has been proposed in the hypothesis of humidifying and warming of inhaled air through the nasal passage.

The alteration in nasal fractional exhaled NO (nasal FENO) levels has been described previously in various diseases such as allergic rhinitis (AR), primary ciliary dyskinesia (PCD), cystic fibrosis, and sinusitis [5–8]. Therefore, the measure of nasal FENO is now considered a useful biomarker in clinical practice for patients with rhino-sinusitis diseases. In patients with PCD, nasal FENO measurement is routinely performed for screening this genetic disorder [9]. In patients with AR, nasal FENO has been used to manage the disease in the same manner as FENO in patients with asthma [10]. The increased iNOS expression and activity due to contact with airborne allergens induces the production of nasal FENO in patients with AR. While the correlation between exhaled NO and lower airway inflammation in asthmatic patients due to eosinophils has been demonstrated, the application of nasal FENO measurement in patients with AR is relatively complex and remains controversial.

Hence, this study was conducted to evaluate (1) the correlation between nasal FENO and anthropometric characteristics, symptoms of AR, and nasal peak flows in children without and with AR; and (2) the cut-off of nasal FENO for diagnosis of AR in symptomatic children.

2. Methods

2.1. Patients

Patients with a diagnosis of AR were included in the current study when they were referred to the Clinical Research Center of Lam Dong Medical College for measuring nasal FENO and a skin-prick test. The present study was approved by the IRB of Lam Dong Medical College, Dalat, Vietnam (ID: CDYTLD.NCKH.03.2018); signed written informed consent was obtained from all the study subjects. The study followed the principles of the 1964 Declaration of Helsinki.

2.1.1. Inclusion Criteria

Patients <18 years old with AR symptoms (nasal congestion, runny nose, nasal itching, or sneezing) lasting more than 4 days per week and for more than 4 consecutive weeks were classified into the AR group.

2.1.2. Exclusion Criteria

The exclusion criteria were one of the following features: severe cardiorespiratory disease, AR treated with oral or local corticosteroids, septal deviation or nasal polyp diagnosed, and upper or lower airway infection in the past 15 days; subjects unable to undergo the functional laboratory testing were also excluded from the present study.

2.2. Methods

This was a cross-sectional and descriptive study. All clinical and functional parameters were recorded for analysis. Included study subjects were divided into 2 groups: a control group consisting of healthy people without nasal and sinus diseases, and the AR group consisting of patients who met the selection criteria.

The criteria for a diagnosis of AR were: having one of the symptoms of nasal congestion, nasal itching and sneezing, and a runny nose lasting more than 4 days/week according to the season or occurring when exposed to respiratory allergens (dog or cat fur, pollen, mold, and house dust mites) in the living or working environment [11].

2.2.1. Laboratory Functional Testing

The peak inspiratory and expiratory flows (PIF and PEF) in the nose were measured by using a nasal mask-attached peak-flow meter device (Mediflux, Bry Sur Marne, France). Nasal FENO measurement was performed by using multi-flow exhaled NO (Hypair NO,

Medisoft; B-5503 Sorinnes; Belgium). Nasal FENO measurement was carried out according to the manufacturer's instructions.

2.2.2. Statistical Analyses

SPSS 22.0 software (Chicago, IL, USA) was used to analyze all the collected data. Categorical variables are presented as numbers or percentages. Continuous parameters are presented as means ± standard deviation (SD). The skewness–kurtosis test measured the normal distribution. The Mann–Whitney U test was used for the comparison of means between groups. The correlation between nasal FENO and quantitative variables with normal distribution was examined by regression analysis. A p-value < 0.05 was considered statistically significant.

3. Results

From January 2018 to December 2019, 100 subjects participated in the study, including 32 healthy people (control group) and 68 patients diagnosed with AR (AR group). The latter met the selection criteria and performed all the required functional tests.

3.1. Clinical and Functional Characteristics Study Subjects

There was no significant difference between the AR group and control group regarding age, gender, height, weight, and BMI ($p > 0.05$; Table 1). The proportion of AR patients who had symptoms of blocked nose, nasal itching or sneezing, and runny nose was 97%, 100%, and 100%, respectively (Table 1). Peak inspiratory and expiratory volumes in patients with AR were significantly lower than in the control group ($p < 0.01$ and $p < 0.01$; Table 1). The mean nasal FENO was considerably higher in the AR group than in the control group (985 ± 232 ppb vs. 229 ± 155 ppb; $p < 0.001$; Table 1).

Table 1. Clinical and functional characteristics of study subjects.

Characteristics	All Study Subjects	Patients with AR	Control Subjects	p *
Number, subjects (%)	100 (100.0)	68 (68.0)	32 (32.0)	-
Age, years	14 ± 3 (6–17)	14 ± 3 (6–17)	13 ± 4 (6–17)	>0.05
Sex, male/female	1.5	1.6	1.4	>0.05
Height, cm	135 ± 33 (99–169)	134 ± 35 (99–169)	136 ± 31 (105–167)	>0.05
Weight, kg	37 ± 19 (18–57)	37 ± 18 (18–55)	38 ± 19 (19–57)	>0.05
BMI, kg/m²	16.8 ± 3.3	16.7 ± 3.4	16.9 ± 3.2	>0.05
Symptoms of AR				
Blocked nose, %	NA	97.0	0.0	NA
Itching and sneezing, %	NA	100.0	0.0	NA
Running nose, %	NA	100.0	0.0	NA
Nasal peak flow				
Peak inspiratory flow, L/min	72 ± 22	67 ± 14	98 ± 26	<0.01
Peak expiratory flow, L/min	107 ± 23	93 ± 24	124 ± 22	<0.01
Nasal FENO, ppb	618 ± 395 (124–1385)	985 ± 232 (526–1385)	229 ± 65 (152–299)	<0.001

p *: different between AR group and control group; AR: allergic rhinitis; BMI: body mass index; FENO: fractional exhaled nitric oxide; L: liter; ppb: parts per billion; NA: not applicable.

3.2. Correlation between Nasal FENO and the Anthropometric Characteristics of the Control Subjects and Clinical Symptoms in Patients with AR

There was no significant correlation between nasal FENO and the anthropometric characteristics of the control subjects participating in the present study (N = 32; Table 2). Nasal FENO had a significant mild to moderate correlation with clinical symptoms of AR, including blocked nose, itching or sneezing, and runny nose (R = 0.356, 0.679 and 0.587; $p < 0.001$, 0.0001 and 0.001, respectively; N = 68; Table 2).

Table 2. Correlation between nasal FENO and the anthropometric characteristics of the control subjects and with clinical symptoms in patients with AR.

Correlation	Anthropometric Parameters (Control Subjects; N = 32)					Symptoms of AR (AR Patients; N = 68)		
Nasal FENO	Age	Sex	Height	Weight	BMI	Blocked Nose	Itching or Sneezing	Runny Nose
R	0.098	0.325	0.094	0.082	0.076	0.356	0.679	0.587
P	0.124	0.079	0.141	0.325	0.328	0.001	0.0001	0.001

AR: allergic rhinitis; BMI: body mass index; FENO: fractional exhaled nitric oxide.

3.3. Correlation between Nasal FENO and Nasal Peak Flow of Study Subjects

There was no significant correlation between nasal FENO and inspiratory and expiratory peak flow in subjects without AR (control subjects; Table 3). There was a significant and negative linear correlation between nasal FENO and peak inspiratory flow (R = −0.462; $p = 0.0012$; Table 3, Figure 1a) and peak expiratory flow (R = −0.378; $p = 0.0016$; Table 3, Figure 1b).

Table 3. Correlation between nasal FENO and nasal peak flow of study subjects.

Correlation	Control Subjects (N = 32)		AR Patients (N = 68)	
Nasal FENO	Peak Inspiratory Flow	Peak Expiratory Flow	Peak Inspiratory Flow	Peak Expiratory Flow
R	0.095	0.074	−0.462	−0.378
P	0.324	0.417	0.0012	0.0016

AR: allergic rhinitis; FENO: fractional exhaled nitric oxide.

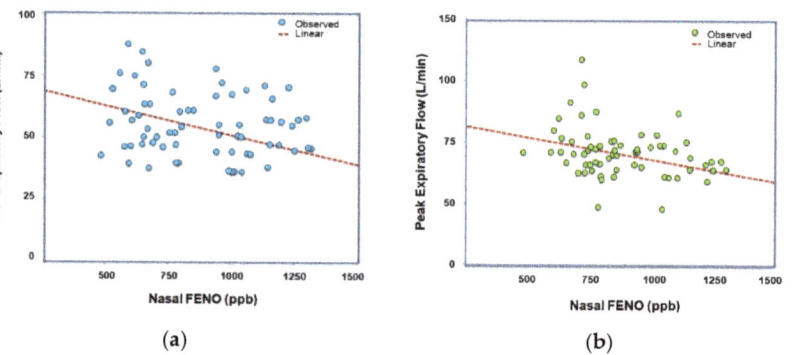

Figure 1. (a) Correlation between nasal FENO and peak inspiratory flow in patients with AR. (b) Correlation between nasal FENO and peak expiratory flow in patients with AR. AR: allergic rhinitis; FENO: fractional exhaled nitric oxide.

3.4. Cut-Off of Nasal FENO in the Diagnosis of AR in Children

The cut-off of nasal FENO in positive diagnoses of AR is presented in Figure 2 and Table 4 (N = 100). The results of ROC curve analysis showed that the cut-off of FENO with the highest Youden index was equivalent to the most significant area under the ROC curve of 794 ppb and had a specificity and sensitivity of 96.7% and 92.6%, respectively. (Figure 2, Table 4).

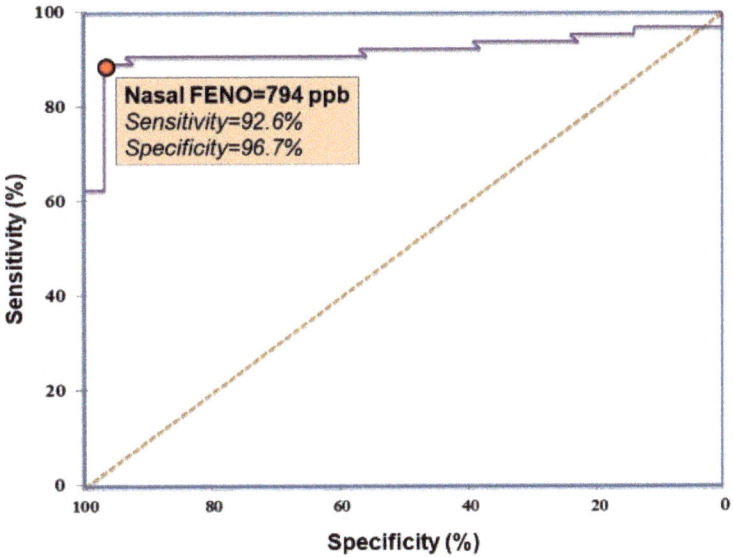

Figure 2. ROC curve of the nasal FENO cut-off for the diagnosis of AR. AR: allergic rhinitis; FENO: fractional exhaled nitric oxide.

Table 4. Cut-off nasal FENO with corresponding AR diagnosis sensitivity and specificity.

Nasal FENO Cut-Off (ppb)	Sensitivity (%)	Specificity (%)	Youden Index
732	94.2	77.3	172.189
738	94.2	81.2	176.213
740	94.2	83.3	178.431
744	94.2	86.1	180.346
749	94.2	89.0	183.890
754	93.7	93.2	187.465
760	92.4	93.1	186.767
794	92.6	96.7	189.234
863	91.7	95.6	188.673
899	91.4	95.6	188.348
905	90.2	95.6	187.560
916	89.8	95.6	186.134
938	88.2	95.6	185.778
945	88.1	95.6	184.657

4. Discussion

The results of our study demonstrated that: (1) Nasal FENO did not depend on anthropometric characteristics or nasal peak inspiratory or expiratory flows in children without AR; (2) there was a correlation between nasal FENO and clinical symptoms, nasal peak inspiratory, and expiratory flows in children with AR; and (3) the cut-off nasal FENO for a diagnosis of AR with the highest specificity and sensitivity was $\geq$794 ppb.

In healthy people, FENO concentrations in the nose are often much higher than in the lower respiratory tract (300–800 ppb vs. 5–25 ppb). In the rhino-sinusal area, the paranasal sinuses are a vital source of nasal FENO production. Previously, Lundberg et al. [8] described that after perforation of the maxillary sinus, the continuous synthesis of NO at a very high concentration was detected. However, Hood et al. [12] showed that only NO concentrations measured in the nasal cavity came from the sinuses by diffusion due to the NO concentration difference between the nose and sinuses, but it was also produced in the nasal cavity. In the present study, the level of nasal FENO in children without AR symptoms was varied from 152 to 298 ppb (Table 1). This result is also consistent with the manufacturer's recommendation that the expected value of nasal FENO in children is less than 300 ppb.

The present study showed that, in control children, the level of nasal FENO was not correlated with anthropometric characteristics such as age, gender, height, weight, and BMI (Table 2). Thus, this is a prominent advantage of nasal FENO as a biomarker because it can be used to diagnose various pathological conditions of the nose regardless of demographic features. It might also be similar to bronchial FENO because a previous study also showed that bronchial FENO had no significant correlation with demographic characteristics [13]. However, the recommended cut-off of the normal value of nasal FENO has been established based on a large population that is representative and takes the age into account [14]. The present study only used a control group with a small sample size to determine the nasal FENO value in healthy children compared with AR children.

Because of the short half-life of NO in gas form, indirect methods were previously used to measure the NO concentration in the body during the humoral phase, based on the measurement of NO metabolism products such as nitrate and nitrite, or using immunohistochemistry techniques to determine NOS activity. In contrast to NO produced in tissue or the blood, exhaled NO in the airways is more stable, allowing us to measure it directly [15–17]. Various techniques have been used to measure exhaled NO concentration, and the most commonly used is the chemiluminescence method. This method is highly sensitive, and exhaled NO can be detected at levels as low as parts per trillion. A new NO analysis method based on the electroluminescence technique has been developed and used in clinical practice (Figure 3) [3,18]. This technique has been shown to have high accuracy and good correlation with other methods, and has the advantage of being small compared with fixed routine chemiluminescence analyzers.

The present study results showed that nasal FENO in children with AR was significantly higher than in children without AR (Table 1). Especially in patients with AR, there was a significant correlation between nasal FENO and clinical symptoms (Table 2). In addition, the results also showed that there was a negative and significant correlation between nasal FENO and nasal peak flows (Table 3 and Figure 1a,b). Obviously, exhaled NO concentration is inversely proportional to the airflow rate. FENO measured in healthy subjects with a flow rate of 50 mL/s had a bronchial FENO level of 5–20 ppb, whereas alveolar FENO (CANO) measured at a flow rate of 150–350 mL/s had a concentration of FENO less than 5 ppb [19]. In the present study, nasal FENO was measured with a HypairNO device by the aspirating method with a constant flow over time. However, the application of nasal NO measurement in subjects with AR is relatively complex because some authors have shown that nasal FENO could be changed after allergen exposure. Definitely, Ragab et al. [12] reported that nasal FENO, but not oral FENO, was significantly increased in patients with seasonal AR during the pollen season. However, Palm et al. [13] reported no change in nasal NO concentration in patients with AR. It is noteworthy that in almost all studies where comorbid sinus disease was excluded, patients with AR had higher nasal NO concentrations compared with healthy subjects. This suggests that there are probably two opposed levels that can determine nasal FENO in patients with RA: firstly, NO gas released from the allergic inflammatory nasal mucosa may be increased although the nasal mucosa are swollen at the same time due to the process of inflammation; secondly, the swollen nasal mucosa might lead to blocked nostrils (ostia) and reduce the flow of NO going out of the nasal cavity, where nasal FENO will be measured.

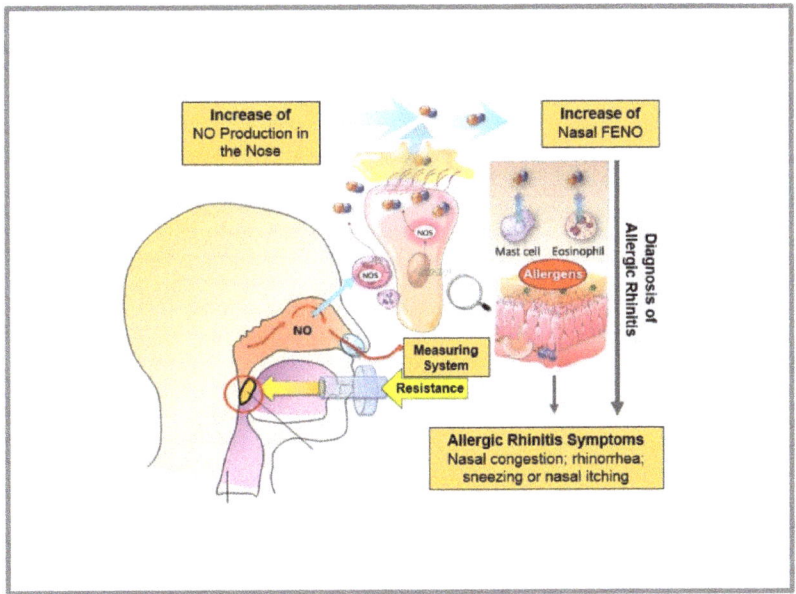

Figure 3. Principle of nasal FENO measurement in subjects with AR [3]. AR: allergic rhinitis; FENO: fractional exhaled nitric oxide; NOS: nitric oxide synthase.

The present study's results showed that the nasal FENO cut-off for a positive diagnosis of AR of 794 ppb was the best diagnostic value (Figure 2, Table 4). The results of ROC curve analysis demonstrated that the cut-off of FENO with the highest Youden index was equivalent to the most significant area under the ROC curve of 794 ppb and had a specificity and sensitivity of 96.7% and 92.6%, respectively (Figure 2 and Table 4). However, the sample size of the present study is not large enough to define the nasal FENO cut-off of a large-scale representative population and for subjects with AR associated with other rhino-sinus comorbidities. This issue is also a main limitation of the present study. Therefore, it is necessary to conduct more studies on nasal FENO in subjects with AR for having reference values in the future.

5. Conclusions

Nasal FENO is a potential biomarker in the diagnosis of allergic rhinitis. The measure of nasal FENO is a simple, low-cost, and non-invasive technique. In addition to the use of nasal FENO in the management of patients with allergic rhinitis, nasal FENO might be used for screening patients with sinusitis, nasal polyps, primary cilliar dyskinesia, and Covid-19 infection. Hence, more studies in patients with these conditions are needed in clinical practice to clarify the role of exhaled NO as a relevant biomarker of non-infectious or viral inflammation.

Author Contributions: Conceptualization, S.D.-Q., T.N.-T.-D., T.N.-V., V.N.-N., L.H.-T. and T.C.; methodology, S.D.-Q., T.N.-T.-D., K.T.-Q., T.T.-T.-T., T.V.-P.-M., Q.V.-T.-T., K.B.-D., V.N.-N., L.H.-T. and T.C.; software, S.D.-Q., T.N.-T.-D., T.T.-T.-T. and T.N.-V.; validation, S.D.-Q., T.N.-T.-D., T.T.-T.-T., Q.V.-T.-T., K.B.-D., V.N.-N. and T.C.; formal analysis, S.D.-Q., T.N.-T.-D., K.T.-Q., T.T.-T.-T., T.N.-V., Q.V.-T.-T. and L.H.-T.; investigation, S.D.-Q., T.N.-T.-D., T.T.-T.-T. and T.N.-V.; resources, S.D.-Q., T.N.-T.-D., K.T.-Q., T.T.-T.-T. and T.N.-V.; data curation, S.D.-Q., T.N.-T.-D., T.T.-T.-T. and T.N.-V.; writing—original draft preparation, S.D.-Q., T.N.-T.-D., Q.V.-T.-T., K.B.-D., V.N.-N. and L.H.-T.; writing—review and editing, S.D.-Q., T.N.-T.-D., Q.V.-T.-T., K.B.-D., V.N.-N., L.H.-T., T.C.; Visualization, S.D.-Q., T.N.-T.-D., T.T.-T.-T., T.N.-V., K.B.-D., V.N.-N.; Supervision, S.D.-Q., T.N.-T.-D., T.T.-T.-T., T.N.-V., L.H.-T. and T.C.; project administration, S.D.-Q., T.T.-T.-T., T.N.-V. and T.C.; funding acquisition, S.D.-Q., T.N.-T.-D., K.T.-Q., T.T.-T.-T. and T.N.-V. All authors have read and agreed to the published version of the manuscript.

Funding: This research received no external funding.

Institutional Review Board Statement: The study was conducted according to the guidelines of the Declaration of Helsinki, and approved by the Institutional Review Board of Lam Dong Medical College (NCKH2018_TTYS_04.18).

Informed Consent Statement: Informed consent was obtained from all subjects involved in the study. Written informed consent has been obtained from the patient(s) to publish this paper.

Conflicts of Interest: The authors declare no conflict of interest.

References

1. Weschta, M.; Deutschle, T.; Riechelmann, H. Nasal fractional exhaled nitric oxide analysis with a novel hand-held device. *Rhinol. J.* **2008**, *46*, 23–27.
2. Bommarito, L.; Guida, G.; Heffler, E.; Badiu, I.; Nebiolo, F.; Usai, A.; De Stefani, A.; Rolla, G. Nasal nitric oxide concentration in suspected chronic rhinosinusitis. *Ann. Allergy Asthma Immunol.* **2008**, *101*, 358–362. [CrossRef]
3. Duong-Quy, S. Clinical Utility Of The Exhaled Nitric Oxide (NO) Measurement With Portable Devices In The Management Of Allergic Airway Inflammation And Asthma. *J. Asthma Allergy* **2019**, *12*, 331–341. [CrossRef] [PubMed]
4. Zysman-Colman, Z.N.; Kaspy, K.R.; Alizadehfar, R.; Nykamp, K.R.; Zariwala, M.A.; Knowles, M.R.; Vinh, D.C.; Shapiro, A.J. Nasal Nitric Oxide in Primary Immunodeficiency and Primary Ciliary Dyskinesia: Helping to Distinguish Between Clinically Similar Diseases. *J. Clin. Immunol.* **2019**, *39*, 216–224. [CrossRef] [PubMed]
5. Mahut, B.; Escudier, E.; De Blic, J.; Zerah-Lancner, F.; Coste, A.; Harf, A.; Delclaux, C. Impairment of Nitric Oxide Output of Conducting Airways in Primary Ciliary Dyskinesia. *Pediatr. Pulmonol.* **2006**, *41*, 158–163. [CrossRef] [PubMed]
6. Degano, B.; Génestal, M.; Serrano, E.; Rami, J.; Arnal, J.-F. Effect of Treatment on Maxillary Sinus and Nasal Nitric Oxide Concentrations in Patients With Nosocomial Maxillary Sinusitis. *Chest* **2005**, *128*, 1699–1705. [CrossRef] [PubMed]
7. Seidman, M.D.; Gurgel, R.K.; Lin, S.Y.; Schwartz, S.R.; Baroody, F.M.; Bonner, J.R.; Dawson, D.E.; Dykewicz, M.S.; Hackell, J.M.; Han, J.K.; et al. Clinical practice guideline: Allergic rhinitis executive summary. *Otolaryngol Head Neck Surg.* **2015**, *152*, 197–206. [CrossRef] [PubMed]
8. Lundberg, J.O.N.; Farkas-Szallasi, T.; Weitzberg, E.; Rinder, J.; Lidholm, J.; Änggård, A.; Hökfelt, T.; Alving, K. High nitric oxide production in human paranasal sinuses. *Nat. Med.* **1995**, *1*, 370–373. [CrossRef] [PubMed]
9. Shapiro, A.J.; Dell, S.D.; Gaston, B.; O'Connor, M.; Marozkina, N.; Manion, M.; Hazucha, M.J.; Leigh, M.W. Nasal Nitric Oxide Measurement in Primary Ciliary Dyskinesia. A Technical Paper on Standardized Testing Protocols. *Ann. Am. Thorac. Soc.* **2020**, *17*, e1–e12. [CrossRef] [PubMed]
10. Vo-Thi-Kim, A.; Van-Quang, T.; Nguyen-Thanh, B.; Dao-Van, D.; Duong-Quy, S. The effect of medical treatment on nasal exhaled nitric oxide (NO) in patients with persistent allergic rhinitis: A randomized control study. *Adv. Med. Sci.* **2020**, *65*, 182–188. [CrossRef] [PubMed]
11. Bousquet, J.; Schünemann, H.J.; Hellings, P.; Arnavielhe, S.; Bachert, C.; Bedbrook, A.; Bergmann, K.-C.; Bosnic-Anticevich, S.; Brozek, J.; Calderon, M.; et al. MACVIA clinical decision algorithm in adolescents and adults with allergic rhinitis. *J. Allergy Clin. Immunol.* **2016**, *138*, 367–374.e2. [CrossRef] [PubMed]
12. Hood, C.M.; Schroter, R.C.; Doorly, D.J.; Blenke, E.J.S.M.; Tolley, N.S. Computational modeling of flow and gas exchange in models of the human maxillary sinus. *J. Appl. Physiol.* **2009**, *107*, 1195–1203. [CrossRef] [PubMed]
13. Pham Van, L.; Duong-Quy, S. Reference values of FENO in respiratory diseases: First large-scale study in Vietnam. *J. Funct. Vent. Pulmonol.* **2014**, *5*. [CrossRef]
14. Society, A.T.; Society, E.R. ATS/ERS Recommendations for Standardized Procedures for the Online and Offline Measurement of Exhaled Lower Respiratory Nitric Oxide and Nasal Nitric Oxide, 2005. *Am. J. Respir. Crit. Care Med.* **2005**, *171*, 912–930. [CrossRef]
15. Duong-Quy, S.; Hua-Huy, T.; Tran-Mai-Thi, H.-T.; Le-Dong, N.-N.; Craig, T.J.; Dinh-Xuan, A.T. Study of Exhaled Nitric Oxide in Subjects with Suspected Obstructive Sleep Apnea: A Pilot Study in Vietnam. *Pulm. Med.* **2016**, *2016*, 1–7. [CrossRef] [PubMed]

16. Hoang-Duc, H.; Pham-Huy, Q.; Vu-Minh, T.; Duong-Quy, S. Study of the Correlation between HRCT Semi-quantitative Scoring, Concentration of Alveolar Nitric Oxide, and Clinical-functional Parameters of Systemic Sclerosis-induced Interstitial Lung Disease. *Yale J. Biol. Med.* **2020**, *93*, 657–667. [PubMed]
17. Duong-Quy, S.; Ngo-Minh, X.; Tang-Le-Quynh, T.; Tang-Thi-Thao, T.; Nguyen-Quoc, B.; Le-Quang, K.; Tran-Thanh, D.; Doan-Thi-Quynh, N.; Canty, E.; Do, T.; et al. The use of exhaled nitric oxide and peak expiratory flow to demonstrate improved breathability and antimicrobial properties of novel face mask made with sustainable filter paper and Folium Plectranthii amboinicii oil: Additional option for mask shortage during COVID-19 pandemic. *Multidiscip. Respir. Med.* **2020**, *15*, 664. [CrossRef] [PubMed]
18. Duong-Quy, S.; Le-Thi-Minh, H.; Nguyen-Thi-Bich, H.; Pham-Thu, H.; Thom, V.; Pham-Thi-Hong, N.; Duong-Thi-Ly, H.; Nguyen-Huy, B.; Ngo-Minh, X.; Nguyen-Thi-Dieu, T.; et al. Correlations between exhaled nitric oxide, rs28364072 polymorphism of FCER2 gene, asthma control, and inhaled corticosteroid responsiveness in children with asthma. *J. Breath Res.* **2020**, *15*, 016012. [CrossRef] [PubMed]
19. Dang-Thi-Mai, K.; Le-Dong, N.-N.; Le-Thuong, V.; Tran-Van, N.; Duong-Quy, S. Exhaled Nitric Oxide as a Surrogate Marker for Obstructive Sleep Apnea Severity Grading: An In-Hospital Population Study. *Nat. Sci. Sleep* **2021**, *13*, 763–773. [CrossRef] [PubMed]

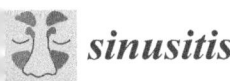

Review

Olfactory Disorders in Post-Acute COVID-19 Syndrome

Laura Araújo [1], Vanessa Arata [1] and Ricardo G. Figueiredo [1,2,3,*]

[1] Departamento de Saúde, Universidade Estadual de Feira de Santana (UEFS), Feira de Santana 44036-900, Brazil; laurabeatrizars@hotmail.com (L.A.); vafigueiredo@uefs.br (V.A.)
[2] Fundação ProAR, Salvador 41940-455, Brazil
[3] Programa de Pós-Graduação em Saúde Coletiva, Universidade Estadual de Feira de Santana (UEFS), Feira de Santana 44036-900, Brazil
* Correspondence: rgfigueiredo@uefs.br

Abstract: Altered smell is one of the most prevalent symptoms in acute COVID-19 infection. Although most patients recover normal neurosensory function in a few weeks, approximately one-tenth of patients report long-term smell dysfunction, including anosmia, hyposmia, parosmia and phantosmia, with a particularly notable impact on quality of life. In this complex scenario, inflammation and cellular damage may play a key role in the pathogenesis of olfactory dysfunctions and may affect olfactory signaling from the peripheral to the central nervous system. Appropriate management of smell disturbances in COVID-19 patients must focus on the underlying mechanisms and the assessment of neurosensorial pathways. This article aims to review the aspects of olfactory impairment, including its pathophysiology, epidemiology, and clinical management in post-acute COVID-19 syndrome (PACS).

Keywords: olfactory dysfunction; anosmia; post-acute COVID-19

1. Introduction

Coronavirus 2019 (COVID-19) disease emerged in Wuhan, China, and has subsequently spread worldwide. The pathological agent of COVID-19 is severe acute respiratory syndrome coronavirus 2 (SARS-CoV-2), an enveloped positive single-stranded RNA virus. COVID-19 is a highly transmissible illness with a broad spectrum of clinical manifestations and variable severity degrees depending on age, comorbidities, genetic factors, and basal metabolic index [1,2]. Individuals may present with a wide range of symptoms, including fatigue, headache, difficulty breathing, diarrhea, nausea, vomiting, loss of taste and smell, runny nose, and muscle and body ache, often indistinguishable from most respiratory viral infections [3].

COVID-19 can induce abnormalities in taste and smell perception, in both the acute and chronic phases of the disease. Smell disturbances are described as: anosmia—a total absence of smell; hyposmia—a diminished sense of smell; parosmia—distorted perception of an existing odor; and phantosmia—perception of smell when no odor source is present. These neurosensory changes have a pronounced impact on quality of life, as most experiences are malodorous, particularly in the qualitative dysfunctions (parosmia and phantosmia) [4].

Angiotensin-converting enzyme-2 receptors (ACE-2) and transmembrane protease serine 2 (TMPRSS2), expressed in the cells of the nasal epithelium, are known pathways for SARS-CoV-2 entry to the respiratory system [5]. Inflammation and cellular damage may play a key role in the pathogenesis of qualitative olfactory dysfunctions. After its internalization, the virus induces an inflammatory response, undergoing maturation and replication inside the cell, as well as involving the recruitment of immune cells [6,7]. SARS-CoV-2 can trigger an unbalanced immune response which overloads the targeted tissues with cytokines and T-cell mediated inflammation [6,7]. The damage caused by the latter may affect olfactory signaling from the peripheral to the central nervous system [8,9].

While most survivors will experience a full recovery, follow-up reveals that a high proportion of individuals still report symptoms after the clearance of the acute infection. The terms 'long COVID' (>4 weeks) as well as 'post-acute COVID' (>3 weeks) and 'chronic COVID' (>12 weeks) have been used to describe these ongoing symptoms [8,10].

2. Epidemiology

Accumulating evidence indicates that altered smell is one of the most prevalent symptoms in acute COVID-19 infection [11]. In self-report studies, the estimated prevalence of olfactory disorders in acute COVID-19 ranged from 5% to 85%, depending on disease severity, and seems to be higher than in other respiratory viral infections. Although most of the patients recover normal neurosensory function in a few weeks, approximately one-tenth of patients reported long-term smell dysfunction, including anosmia, hyposmia, parosmia and phantosmia, with a particularly notable impact on quality of life [12].

Qualitative olfactory dysfunctions are often undervalued in the clinical management of COVID-19 infection and are generally underestimated in observational self-report studies. Individuals may experience a range of persistent and prolonged olfactory sequelae in PACS (Table 1). Continued loss of smell after several weeks was reported in 1.7–29% of patients with COVID-19 requiring hospitalization [13–16]. Disturbed taste and smell were also prevalent after 6 months in approximately one quarter of home-isolated young adults with a milder course of the disease [17]. In a cohort of 467 patients in the United Kingdom followed up at 4–6 weeks, participants with positive SARS-CoV-2 IgM/IgG antibodies reported significantly higher prevalence of longstanding smell loss compared to participants with a negative antibody test, with rates of full resolution of olfactory impairment of 57.7% and 72.1%, respectively [18]. In addition, female individuals were almost 2.5 times more likely to experience persistent smell loss compared to participants of the male sex, and parosmia was also significantly associated with unresolved smell loss at 4 to 6 weeks follow-up [18].

3. Pathophysiogenesis of Olfactory Dysfunction

SARS-CoV-2's route of infection basically comprises two pathways: through cell entry factors such as angiotensin-converting enzyme 2 (ACE2), transmembrane protease serine 2 (TMPRSS2), and furin, or through an endosomal route that does not require previous cleavage of the spike protein (S). ACE2 can act as a primary receptor, and, after virus attachment, the spike protein in its surface is cleaved and dissociated by furin, after which the subunit S2 is cleaved by TMPRSS2, changing the structure of the S2 subunit, which ultimately leads to membrane fusion and viral RNA transferring to host cell cytoplasm. An alternative pathway can also be initiated by ACE2 binding and the internalization process involving clathrin and cathepsin L, and, in this case, the virus releases its genetic material directly after endocytosis, as an alternative independent from TMPRSS2 to invade cells [19].

After entering the mouth through salivary particles, the virus can infect cells in filiform and vallate papillae, lingual epithelium and taste buds, all cells that express ACE2, starting its replication, which in turn causes taste impairment [19]. Other potential targets for cell infection due to ACE2 are vascular endothelial cells and adipocytes in parotid and salivary glands. The damage in these cells affects both blood and nutritional supplies and, indirectly, it can change taste perception [19].

Upper airway mucosa has nasal goblet and ciliated cells expressing ACE2 and TMPRSS2, and these respiratory epithelium cell types may have a role in facilitating SARS-CoV-2 infection by storing viral particles [20].

High levels of ACE2 were found in sustentacular cells of the olfactory system, which are in intimate contact with dendrites of olfactory receptor neurons, and also other olfactory epithelium cells such as ductal cells of Bowman's gland, microvillar cells, globose and horizontal basal cells, and olfactory bulb pericytes [19,21]. It is hypothesized that infection of mesenchymal stromal and vascular cells in the nose and bulb and their subsequent inflammation affects the neuronal conduction, reduces nutritional and water supplies and, therefore, causes the death of olfactory sensory neurons (OSNs) and damage to olfactory bulb function [20] (Figure 1). Although OSNs are surprisingly not an ACE2 expressing tissue, it has already been described that the spike protein can bind to neural cell receptors, possibly due to cell-to-cell transmission through tunneling nanotubes (TNTs), filamentous cellular projections that form a communication and transportation net between cells [19].

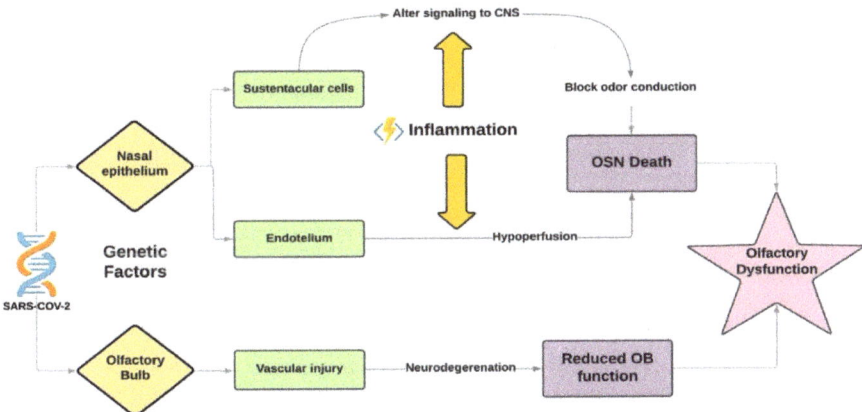

Figure 1. Pathogenesis of olfactory dysfunction. Infection of mesenchymal stromal and vascular cells in the nose and bulb and their subsequent inflammation affect the neuronal conduction, reduce nutritional and water supplies and, therefore, cause the death of olfactory sensory neurons (OSNs) and damage to olfactory bulb function. SARS-COV-2 indicates severe acute respiratory syndrome coronavirus 2; CNS, central nervous system; OB, olfactory bulb; OSN, olfactory sensory neurons.

Neuropilin-1 represents another host factor that facilitates SARS-CoV-2 entry, and its presence was detected in mitral cells of the olfactory bulb, but not in the OE, and the virus may enter the central nervous system (CNS) through retrograde axonal transport from the nasal cavity in a process mediated by ACE2, TMPRSS2 and nicotinic receptors [22]. SARS-CoV-2 uses olfactory neurons to approach the CNS, and similar mechanisms were described for SARS-CoV-1, MERS-CoV, and HCoV-OCR43. The neuronal damage in axons, the death of neurons and microhemorrhages in the bulb may extend the period of smell disturbances [22].

To sum up, these are the ways through which SARS-CoV-2 may cause olfactory dysfunction: conductive dysfunction, by mechanically blocking smell from reaching neuroepithelium; sensorineural dysfunction by attacking directly or indirectly olfactory neuroepithelium or OSNs; and central dysfunction, by affecting bulb neurons [22].

4. Smell Dysfunction in PACS

Smell dysfunction can occur in the context of various infectious viral diseases [23]. Alteration of smell can be categorized into two distinct types: quantitative and qualitative, and subcategorized in total/complete or partial/incomplete, as well as in unilateral or bilateral [23]. Quantitative loss is seen in anosmia and hyposmia, while qualitative loss is noted in parosmia and phantosmia [24].

Anosmia and hyposmia can be assessed by running olfactory tests such as "le nez du vin" or "scratch and sniff" pads containing variable odorant samples [23,25]. Notably, hyposmia and anosmia in infectious diseases are distinguished from nasal inflammation by their lack of seasonal variance, and sometimes permanent length of stay [23].

In contrast to common upper airways infection, rhinorrhea or nasal congestion are less associated with anosmia in COVID-19; however, it can affect the central nervous system, as observed in an 18-FDG PET/CT study, in which a reduction in metabolic activity was reported in the left orbitofrontal cortex, and it can be associated with edema of the olfactory bulb in MRI [26–28]. Anosmia can lead to suspicion of COVID-19 diagnosis, as it can be the only clinical feature present [29].

Hyposmia was reported in a study in Padua as an isolated or more prominent symptom of SARS-CoV-2 infection, often associated with hypogeusia [25]. Hyposmia and parosmia can be persistent olfactory dysfunctions in PACS [28].

Parosmia and phantosmia are distortions in smell perception. Parosmia is a disorder in which an odor is perceived as a different smell, either pleasant—euosmia—or unpleasant—troposmia [25]. Troposmia is often referred to as a burned, foul or rotten smell [27]. In an 18-FDG PET/CT study, the activity in the secondary olfactory cortex was preserved in a patient presenting parosmia post anosmia after COVID-19 infection [27]. In another study, reduced olfactory bulb activity was associated with parosmia [27]. Parosmia and anosmia can be related, and loss of smell can evolve into parosmia in the context of SARS-CoV-2 infection [18].

Parosmia can be related to peripheral and central injuries by SARS-CoV-2, since it can affect OSNs and olfactory centers in the bulb [27]. The growth of new olfactory axons can occur in a non-organized manner and, as a consequence, it prolongs parosmia [18]. Data concerning post-infectious parosmia point to a poorer prognostic value towards the recuperation of smell ability, although olfactory training can help in the recovery of smell [18].

In phantosmia, the smell sensation is generated even in the absence of odors [24]. Smell disturbances can affect taste perception [30]. Taste dysfunctions post COVID-19 infection can also be categorized as qualitative or quantitative. Qualitative taste alterations are known as dysgeusia, whereas quantitative ones are referred to as hypogeusia, in which taste is decreased, and ageusia, in which taste sensation is non-existent [20]. The inflammatory response may cause reparable damage to the taste buds, and as a consequence, a short recovery time can be expected. An unbalanced immune response may also be an agent for a bad prognosis in sensory loss, since the T-cell response is present in sialadenitis and xerostomia [20]. Additionally, distortion in chemosensory perception, such as parosmia or dysgeusia, may increase the probability of long-term smell and/or taste loss and longer COVID-19 symptoms [18].

5. Clinical Management Considerations

Despite overcoming systemic inflammation and respiratory distress in the acute phase of COVID-19 infection, some patients present prolonged inflammation and tissue damage. Appropriate management of smell disturbances in COVID-19 patients must focus on the underlying mechanisms and the assessment of neurosensorial pathways. Although most COVID-19-related acute olfactory dysfunctions improve spontaneously, treatment for persistent smell symptoms may be reasonable when impairment lingers beyond 2 weeks [31]. However, the efficacy of available treatment in PACS remains unclear.

Olfactory rehabilitation has been described as an effective method for restoring the sense of smell in post-infectious olfactory dysfunction (PIOD). Olfactory training is a simple and safe strategy defined as repeated and conscious sniffing of a set of odorants, for 15–20 s each, at least twice a day [32]. Additionally, the conscious focus on odors, in addition to human olfactory ecology including social and physical environment triggers, may effectively stimulate the neurosensorial system and enhance olfactory performance [33]. A retrospective German study of 153 patients with PIOD showed clinically relevant improvements in overall quantitative and qualitative function upon receiving olfactory training (OT). Additionally, the presence of parosmia was associated with significant improvement of olfactory performance after OT [34].

Oral and nasal corticosteroids may be used to control a potential inflammatory component in PIOD; however, current evidence does not support the routine administration of systemic corticosteroids in this scenario due to safety concerns. Additionally, unless inflammatory features in endoscopic or imaging evaluation are detected, it is improbable that corticosteroids would be helpful. [31]. A recent randomized controlled trial (RCT) failed to prove the superiority of mometasone furoate topical nasal therapy over OT in the treatment of post COVID-19 anosmia. [35]. Notably, intranasal corticosteroid therapy in patients with allergic rhinitis and concomitant COVID-19 infection have recently been reviewed in an ARIA-EAACI position paper. These have been shown to be safe and should be considered, at the recommended dose, on a case-by-case basis [36].

Table 1. Prevalence of olfactory dysfunction in post-acute COVID-19 syndrome.

Author	Country	Setting	Time (Days)	Population	n	Prevalence of Olfactory/Gustatory Dysfunction
Garrigues 2020 [13]	France	Cross sectional, single center	110.9	Hospitalized	120	Anosmia (13.3%)
Chopra 2020 [14]	United States	Prospective cohort, multicenter	60	Hospitalized	488	Loss of taste and/or smell (28%)
Rosales-Castillo 2020 [15]	Spain	Retrospective cohort, single center	50.8	Hospitalized	118	Anosmia (1.7%)
Jacobs 2020 [16]	United States	Prospective cohort, single center	35	Hospitalized	183	Lack of smell (9.3%)
Daher 2020 [37]	Germany	Prospective cohort, single center	42	Hospitalized	33	Loss of smell (12%)
Klein 2020 [38]	Israel	Prospective cohort, single center	180	Hospitalized (5.5%) and home-isolated	112	Smell changes (9.8%)
Moreno-Pérez 2021 [39]	Spain	Prospective cohort, multicenter	112–126	Hospitalized (58.2%) and home-isolated	277	Anosmia-dysgeusia (21%)
Seessle 2021 [40]	Germany	Prospective cohort, single center	360	Hospitalized (32.3%) and home-isolated	96	Anosmia (20.8%)
Tenford 2020 [41]	United States	Cross sectional, multicenter	14–21	Home-isolated	270	Loss of smell (27%)
Boscolo-Rizzo 2020 [42]	Italy	Cross sectional, single center	28	Home-isolated	187	Altered sense of smell or taste (51.3%)
Paderno 2020 [43]	Italy	Prospective cohort, multicenter	30	Home-isolated	151	Olfactory dysfunction (17.7%)
Valiente-De Santis 2020 [44]	Spain	Prospective cohort, single center	84	Home-isolated	108	Anosmia (9.3%)
Otte 2020 [45]	Germany	Cross sectional, single center	56	Home-isolated	80	Hyposmia (45.1%)
Blomberg 2021 [17]	Norway	Prospective cohort, multicenter	168	Home-isolated	247	Disturbed taste/smell (27%)

COVID-19 indicates coronavirus disease 2019; Time, time to assessment in days; n, sample size.

Author Contributions: L.A., V.A., R.G.F. contributed equally to this work. All authors have read and agreed to the published version of the manuscript.

Funding: This research received no external funding.

Conflicts of Interest: The authors declare no conflict of interest.

References

1. Escandón, K.; Rasmussen, A.L.; Bogoch, I.I.; Murray, E.J.; Escandón, K.; Popescu, S.V.; Kindrachuk, J. COVID-19 false dichotomies and a comprehensive review of the evidence regarding public health, COVID-19 symptomatology, SARS-CoV-2 transmission, mask wearing, and reinfection. *BMC Infect. Dis.* **2021**, *21*, 1–47. [CrossRef]
2. Cevik, M.; Kuppalli, K.; Kindrachuk, J.; Peiris, M. Virology, transmission, and pathogenesis of SARS-CoV-2. *BMJ* **2020**, *371*, 1–6.
3. Centers for Disease Control and Prevention. Interim Clinical Guidance for Management of Patients with Confirmed Coronavirus Disease (COVID-19). Available online: https://www.cdc.gov/coronavirus/2019-ncov/hcp/clinical-guidance-management-patients.html (accessed on 21 August 2021).
4. Keller, A.; Malaspina, D. Hidden consequences of olfactory dysfunction: A patient report series. *BMC Ear Nose Throat Disord.* **2013**, *13*. [CrossRef]
5. Bourgonje, A.R.; Abdulle, A.E.; Timens, W.; Hillebrands, J.L.; Navis, G.J.; Gordijn, S.J.; Bolling, M.C.; Dijkstra, G.; Voors, A.A.; Osterhaus, A.D.; et al. Angiotensin-converting enzyme 2 (ACE2), SARS-CoV-2 and the pathophysiology of coronavirus disease 2019 (COVID-19). *J. Pathol.* **2020**, *251*, 228–248. [CrossRef]
6. Hamming, I.; Timens, W.; Bulthuis, M.L.C.; Lely, A.T.; Navis, G.J.; van Goor, H. Tissue distribution of ACE2 protein, the functional receptor for SARS coronavirus. A first step in understanding SARS pathogenesis. *J. Pathol.* **2004**, *203*, 631–637. [CrossRef] [PubMed]
7. Wu, Z.; McGoogan, J.M. Characteristics of and Important Lessons from the Coronavirus Disease 2019 (COVID-19) Outbreak in China: Summary of a Report of 72314 Cases from the Chinese Center for Disease Control and Prevention. *JAMA J. Am. Med. Assoc.* **2020**, *323*, 1239–1242. [CrossRef] [PubMed]
8. Shah, W.; Hillman, T.; Playford, E.D.; Hishmeh, L. Managing the long term effects of covid-19: Summary of NICE, SIGN, and RCGP rapid guideline. *BMJ* **2021**, *372*, n136. [CrossRef] [PubMed]
9. Tsuchiya, H. Oral symptoms associated with COVID-19 and their pathogenic mechanisms: A literature review. *Dent. J.* **2021**, *9*, 32. [CrossRef] [PubMed]
10. Greenhalgh, T.; Knight, M.; A'Court, C.; Buxton, M.; Husain, L. Management of post-acute covid-19 in primary care. *BMJ* **2020**, *370*, m3026. [CrossRef]
11. Printza, A.; Katotomichelakis, M.; Valsamidis, K.; Metallidis, S.; Panagopoulos, P.; Panopoulou, M.; Petrakis, V.; Constantinidis, J. Smell and Taste Loss Recovery Time in COVID-19 Patients and Disease Severity. *J. Clin. Med.* **2021**, *10*, 966. [CrossRef]
12. Parma, V.; Ohla, K.; Veldhuizen, M.G.; Niv, M.Y.; Kelly, C.E.; Bakke, A.J.; Cooper, K.W.; Bouysset, C.; Pirastu, N.; Dibattista, M. More than smell—COVID-19 is associated with severe impairment of smell, taste, and chemesthesis. *Chem. Senses* **2020**, *45*, 609–622. [CrossRef]
13. Garrigues, E.; Janvier, P.; Kherabi, Y.; Le Bot, A.; Hamon, A.; Gouze, H.; Doucet, L.; Berkani, S.; Oliosi, E.; Mallart, E.; et al. Post-discharge persistent symptoms and health-related quality of life after hospitalization for COVID-19. *J. Infect.* **2020**, *81*, e4–e6. [CrossRef] [PubMed]
14. Chopra, V.; Flanders, S.A.; O'Malley, M.; Malani, A.N.; Prescott, H.C. Sixty-day outcomes among patients hospitalized wed. *Am. J. Physiol. Cell Physiol.* **2020**, *319*, 945.
15. Rosales-Castillo, A.; García de los Ríos, C.; Mediavilla García, J.D. Persistent symptoms after acute COVID-19 infection: Importance of follow-up. *Med. Clínica Engl. Ed.* **2021**, *156*, 35–36.
16. Jacobs, L.G.; Paleoudis, E.G.; Di Bari, D.L.; Nyirenda, T.; Friedman, T.; Gupta, A.; Rasouli, L.; Zetkulic, M.; Balani, B.; Ogedegbe, C.; et al. Persistence of symptoms and quality of life at 35 days after hospitalization for COVID-19 infection. *PLoS ONE* **2020**, *15*, e0243882. [CrossRef] [PubMed]
17. Blomberg, B.; Mohn, K.G.I.; Brokstad, K.A.; Zhou, F.; Linchausen, D.W.; Hansen, B.A.; Lartey, S.; Onyango, T.B.; Kuwelker, K.; Sævik, M.; et al. Long COVID in a prospective cohort of home-isolated patients. *Nat. Med.* **2021**, *23*, 1–7.
18. Makaronidis, J.; Firman, C.; Magee, C.G.; Mok, J.; Balogun, N.; Lechner, M.; Carnemolla, A.; Batterham, R.L. Distorted chemosensory perception and female sex associate with persistent smell and/or taste loss in people with SARS-CoV-2 antibodies: A community based cohort study investigating clinical course and resolution of acute smell and/or taste loss in people. *BMC Infect. Dis.* **2021**, *21*, 221. [CrossRef] [PubMed]
19. Okada, Y.; Yoshimura, K.; Toya, S.; Tsuchimochi, M. Pathogenesis of taste impairment and salivary dysfunction in COVID-19 patients. *Jpn. Dent. Sci. Rev.* **2021**, *57*, 111–122. [CrossRef]
20. Brann, D.H.; Tsukahara, T.; Weinreb, C.; Lipovsek, M.; Van Den Berge, K.; Gong, B.; Chance, R.; Macaulay, I.C.; Chou, H.J.; Fletcher, R.B.; et al. Non-neuronal expression of SARS-CoV-2 entry genes in the olfactory system suggests mechanisms underlying COVID-19-associated anosmia. *Sci. Adv.* **2020**, *6*, eabc5801. [CrossRef]
21. Wang, F.; Kream, R.M.; Stefano, G.B. Long-term respiratory and neurological sequelae of COVID-19. *Med. Sci. Monit.* **2020**, *26*, e928996. [CrossRef] [PubMed]
22. Kapoor, D.; Verma, N.; Gupta, N.; Goyal, A. Post Viral Olfactory Dysfunction After SARS-CoV-2 Infection: Anticipated Post-pandemic Clinical Challenge. *Indian J. Otolaryngol. Head Neck Surg.* **2021**, 1–8. [CrossRef]
23. Doty, R.L. The olfactory system and Its disorders. *Semin Neurol.* **2009**, *29*, 74–81. [CrossRef] [PubMed]
24. Rashid, R.A.; Alaqeedy, A.A.; Al-Ani, R.M. Parosmia Due to COVID-19 Disease: A 268 Case Series. *Indian J. Otolaryngol. Head Neck Surg.* **2021**, 1–8. [CrossRef]

25. Marchese-Ragona, R.; Ottaviano, G.; Piero, N.; Vianello, A.; Miryam, C. Sudden hyposmia as a prevalent symptom of COVID-19 infection. *medRxiv* **2020**. [CrossRef]
26. Guedj, E.; Campion, J.Y.; Dudouet, P.; Kaphan, E.; Bregeon, F.; Tissot-Dupont, H.; Guis, S.; Barthelemy, F.; Habert, P.; Ceccaldi, M.; et al. 18F-FDG brain PET hypometabolism in patients with long COVID. *Eur. J. Nucl. Med. Mol. Imaging* **2021**, *48*, 2823–2833. [CrossRef] [PubMed]
27. Yousefi-Koma, A.; Haseli, S.; Bakhshayeshkaram, M.; Raad, N.; Karimi-Galougahi, M. Multimodality Imaging With PET/CT and MRI Reveals Hypometabolism in Tertiary Olfactory Cortex in Parosmia of COVID-19. *Acad. Radiol.* **2021**, *28*, 749–751. [CrossRef] [PubMed]
28. Xydakis, M.S.; Albers, M.W.; Holbrook, E.H.; Lyon, D.M.; Shih, R.Y.; Frasnelli, J.A.; Pagenstecher, A.; Kupke, A.; Enquist, L.W.; Perlman, S. Post-viral effects of COVID-19 in the olfactory system and their implications. *Lancet Neurol.* **2021**, *20*, 753–761. [CrossRef]
29. Mehraeen, E.; Behnezhad, F.; Salehi, M.A.; Noori, T.; Harandi, H.; SeyedAlinaghi, S.A. Olfactory and gustatory dysfunctions due to the coronavirus disease (COVID-19): A review of current evidence. *Eur. Arch. Oto-Rhino-Laryngol.* **2021**, *278*, 307–312. [CrossRef]
30. Crook, H.; Raza, S.; Nowell, J.; Young, M.; Edison, P. Long covid—Mechanisms, risk factors, and management. *BMJ* **2021**, *374*. [CrossRef]
31. Whitcroft, K.L.; Hummel, T. Olfactory Dysfunction in COVID-19: Diagnosis and Management. *JAMA J. Am. Med. Assoc.* **2020**, *323*, 2512–2514. [CrossRef]
32. Hummel, T.; Reden, K.R.J.; Hähner, A.; Weidenbecher, M.; Hüttenbrink, K.B. Effects of olfactory Training in patients with olfactory loss. *Laryngoscope* **2009**, *119*, 496–499. [CrossRef]
33. Oleszkiewicz, A.; Heyne, L.; Sienkiewicz-Oleszkiewicz, B.; Cuevas, M.; Haehner, A.; Hummel, T. Odours count: Human olfactory ecology appears to be helpful in the improvement of the sense of smell. *Sci. Rep.* **2021**, *11*, 16888. [CrossRef] [PubMed]
34. Liu, D.T.; Sabha, M.; Damm, M.; Philpott, C.; Oleszkiewicz, A.; Hähner, A.; Hummel, T. Parosmia is Associated with Relevant Olfactory Recovery After Olfactory Training. *Laryngoscope* **2021**, *131*, 618–623. [CrossRef] [PubMed]
35. Abdelalim, A.A.; Mohamady, A.A.; Elsayed, R.A.; Elawady, M.A.; Ghallab, A.F. Corticosteroid nasal spray for recovery of smell sensation in COVID-19 patients: A randomized controlled trial. *Am. J. Otolaryngol.* **2021**, *42*, 102884. [CrossRef] [PubMed]
36. Bousquet, J.; Akdis, C.A.; Jutel, M.; Bachert, C.; Klimek, L.; Agache, I.; Ansotegui, I.J.; Bedbrook, A.; Bosnic-Anticevich, S.; Canonica, G.W.; et al. Intranasal corticosteroids in allergic rhinitis in COVID-19 infected patients: An ARIA-EAACI statement. *Allergy Eur. J. Allergy Clin. Immunol.* **2020**, *75*, 2440–2444. [CrossRef] [PubMed]
37. Daher, A.; Balfanz, P.; Cornelissen, C.; Müller, A.; Bergs, I.; Marx, N.; Müller-Wieland, D.; Hartmann, B.; Dreher, M.; Müller, T. Follow up of patients with severe coronavirus disease 2019 (COVID-19): Pulmonary and extrapulmonary disease sequelae. *Respir. Med.* **2020**, *174*, 106197. [CrossRef]
38. Hadar, K.; Kim, A.; Noam, K.; Yuval, B.; Ran, N.P.; Mordechai, M.; Sarah, I.; Masha, Y.N. Onset, duration, and persistence of taste and smell changes and other COVID-19 symptoms: Longitudinal study in Israeli patients. *MedRxiv* **2020**. [CrossRef]
39. Moreno-Pérez, O.; Merino, E.; Leon-Ramirez, J.M.; Andres, M.; Ramos, J.M.; Arenas-Jiménez, J.; Asensio, S.; Sanchez, R.; Ruiz-Torregrosa, P.; Galan, I.; et al. Post-acute COVID-19 syndrome. Incidence and risk factors: A Mediterranean cohort study. *J. Infect.* **2021**, *82*, 378–383. [CrossRef]
40. Seeßle, J.; Waterboer, T.; Hippchen, T.; Simon, J.; Kirchner, M.; Lim, A.; Müller, B.; Merle, U. Persistent symptoms in adult patients one year after COVID-19: A prospective cohort study. *Clin. Infect. Dis.* **2021**. [CrossRef]
41. Tenforde, M.W.; Kim, S.S.; Lindsell, C.J.; Erica, B.R.; Nathan, I.S.; Clark, F.D.; Kevin, W.G.; Heidi, L.E.; Jay, S.S.; Howard, A.S.; et al. Symptom duration and risk factors for delayed return to usual health among outpatients with COVID-19 in a multistate health care systems network—United States, March-June 2020. *MMWR Morb. Mortal Wkly. Rep.* **2020**, *69*, 993–998. [CrossRef]
42. Boscolo-Rizzo, P.; Borsetto, D.; Fabbris, C.; Spinato, G.; Frezza, D.; Menegaldo, A.; Mularoni, F.; Gaudioso, P.; Cazzador, D.; Marciani, S.; et al. Evolution of Altered Sense of Smell or Taste in Patients With Mildly Symptomatic COVID-19. *JAMA Otolaryngol. Head Neck Surg.* **2020**, *146*, 729–732. [CrossRef]
43. Paderno, A.; Mattavelli, D.; Rampinelli, V.; Grammatica, A.; Raffetti, E.; Tomasoni, M.; Gualtieri, T.; Taboni, S.; Zorzi, S.; Del Bon, F.; et al. Olfactor and gustatory outcomes in COVID-19: A prospective evaluation in nonhospitalized subjects. *Otolaryngol.–Head Neck Surg.* **2020**, *163*, 1144–1149. [CrossRef] [PubMed]
44. Lucía, V.D.S.; Inés, P.C.; Beatriz, S.; Gracia, E.G.; Juan, D.R.M.; Antonio, P.; Ignacio, M.G.; Marcial, D.F.; Manuel, C.; Francisco, O.; et al. Clinical and immunoserological status 12 weeks after infection with COVID-19: Prospective observational study. *MedRxiv* **2020**. [CrossRef]
45. Otte, M.S.; Eckel, H.N.C.; Poluschkin, L.; Klussmann, J.P.; Luers, J.C. Olfactory dysfunction in patients after recovering from COVID-19. *Acta Otolaryngol.* **2020**, *140*, 1032–1035. [CrossRef] [PubMed]

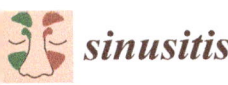 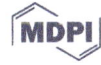

Article

Effects of the Traditional Mediterranean Diet in Childhood Recurrent Acute Rhinosinusitis

Fernando M. Calatayud-Sáez [1,*], Blanca Calatayud [2] and Ana Calatayud [3]

1. Pediatrician at the Child and Adolescent Clinic "La Palma", C/Palma 17, bajo A, 13001 Ciudad Real, Spain
2. Nutritionist at the Child and Adolescent Clinic "La Palma", C/Palma 17, bajo A, 13001 Ciudad Real, Spain; blanca.calatayud@gmail.com
3. Nurse and Nutritionist at the Child and Adolescent Clinic "La Palma", C/Palma 17, bajo A, 13001 Ciudad Real, Spain; anacalatayud94@gmail.com
* Correspondence: altayud1@gmail.com

Abstract: Introduction: There are more and more studies that demonstrate the anti-inflammatory effects of the traditional Mediterranean diet (TMD). The aim of the study was to assess the effects of an intervention with the TMD in patients with recurrent acute and chronic rhinosinusitis. Material and Methods: We performed a pretest–posttest comparison study in 114 patients (56 girls and 58 boys) aged one to five years who had three or more acute rhinosinusitis episodes in the period of 1 year. They were included for a year in the nutritional program "Learning to eat from the Mediterranean". The anthropometric, clinical, and therapeutic characteristics were studied. Results: All the studied indicators showed a positive and statistically significant evolution. Of the patients, 53.5% did not have any episode of acute rhinosinusitis, and 26.3% had only one, compared to the 3.37 they had on average in the previous year. The use of antibiotics decreased by 87.6%. The degree of satisfaction of the families was very high. The Mediterranean Diet Quality Index (KIDMED) that assesses the quality of the TMD rose from 7.7 to 11 points. Conclusions: The adoption of the TMD could have promising effects in the prevention and treatment of recurrent acute and chronic rhinosinusitis, limiting the pharmacological and surgical intervention in many of these patients.

Keywords: acute rhinosinusitis; acute recurrent rhinosinusitis; chronic rhinosinusitis; Mediterranean diet; nutritional evaluation; nutritional therapy

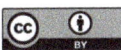

1. Introduction

At the beginning of the school year and with the arrival of winter, young children are prone to illness from upper respiratory tract infections (URTI), which can range between six and eight episodes a year. Most of these colds tend to resolve spontaneously within a week or two. However, 5–10% of patients develop bacterial complications, including acute rhinosinusitis (ARS) and acute otitis media (AOM). It is estimated that between 6% and 13% of children will have had an episode of ARS by three years of age [1,2]. Although it is usually a self-limited disease, it becomes one of the most frequent causes of antibiotic prescription in childhood, behind otitis and tonsillitis [3,4]. ARS is mainly characterized by the excessive prolongation of the symptoms of the common cold beyond 10 days, with difficulty in nasal breathing, mucopurulent discharge, persistent cough predominantly at night, difficulty in falling asleep, loss of appetite, and sometimes vomiting of phlegm [5]. Often there is a spontaneous improvement after conservative treatment with hypertonic saline sprays or irrigations [6]. When the general condition is more affected, or in young children, it may be necessary to use antibiotics [7]. Some patients lengthen the usual colds over and over again, causing recurrent ARS (RARS), which do not usually cause fever, and thus predisposes some parents not to come to the consultation and ends up turning into chronic rhinosinusitis (CRS). They are patients who have persistent green mucus, significant nasal obstruction, difficulty falling asleep and a persistent cough, although with little effect on the general condition. This persistent inflammatory state contributes to the enlargement of the local lymphatic tissue, such as the palatine tonsils and the adenoids, leading to a space conflict [8]. They often present with worsening clinical attacks or other complications, such as recurrent acute otitis media (RAOM), otitis media with effusion (OME), persistent nasal obstruction (PNO) and recurrent wheezing or childhood asthma (SR) [9,10]. The diagnosis of ARS is not straightforward and can be considered as a clinical challenge, as it is generally performed on subtle clinical grounds, with the absence of specific tests. It is difficult to distinguish when a viral process has become bacterial [11]. Routine imaging is not recommended precisely because of its lack of specificity [12–14]. Pharyngeal exudates are also not useful since they do not correlate with sinus exudates. The most common bacterial species are: streptococcus pneumoniae, Hemophilus influenzae, Moraxella catarrhalis, and streptococcus pyogenes [15,16]. The treatment of RARS and CRS is controversial; several types of antibiotics have been used with limited results, since after initial improvement, patients eventually relapse [9,17]. Corticosteroid irrigations through the nasal passages and oral corticosteroids have also been used based on the few studies conducted in children with different results [1,18–20]. Mucolytics, expectorants, and antihistamines have not been shown to be helpful [21,22]. The pneumococcal vaccine does not appear to have decreased the incidence of ARS [13]. In the last case and after having failed with the pharmacological treatment, surgical intervention is usually indicated, with the oblation of the adenoids and/or the palatine tonsils, without the results being entirely satisfactory [23].

There are more and more studies that demonstrate the anti-inflammatory effects of the Mediterranean diet [24], which has allowed us to develop the hypothesis that recurrent inflammatory episodes of the respiratory mucosa are closely related to the abandonment of the traditional diet. This anti-inflammatory action is based on the reduction of pathologies related to oxidative stress, chronic inflammation, and the inflammatory system. Our hypothesis is that diet and individual nutrients can influence the resolution of RARS by stabilizing the inflammatory and immune mechanisms. We have previously conducted studies on the effects of the Mediterranean diet on URTI and their frequent bacterial complications [25], such as recurrent acute otitis media [26], otitis media with effusion [27], persistent nasal obstruction [28], and childhood asthma [29], with satisfactory results. We have also applied the Mediterranean diet in infants since birth and have observed a lower incidence of habitual inflammatory pathology [30]. Following our main line of argument in which we relate recurrent inflammatory episodes with the abandonment of the traditional diet, we have carried out this study on the effects of a traditional Mediterranean diet (TMD) in patients diagnosed with recurrent acute and chronic rhinosinusitis.

2. Material and Methods
2.1. Study Design

The design corresponded to a prospective quasi-experimental study of the comparison of before and after (pre/posttest) of a single group, with each patient examined for one year. The study consecutively included patients aged 1 to 5, diagnosed with RARS and CRS, attending a primary attention pediatrics office between May 2010 and November 2018, with the informed consent of the parents or legal guardians. This study was carried out in the Mediterranean area, in the community of Castilla la Mancha (Spain).

Patients with anatomical abnormalities, allergies, or who had been treated surgically were excluded from the study. The study consisted of comparing the incidence of RARS and CRS in the previous and subsequent years after applying the TMD. The intervention focused on food re-education based on the TMD through the use of the nutritional education program "Learning to eat from the Mediterranean", which was used in previous studies [12,13]. This program consists of a series of visits with the nutritionist and the pediatrician, who propose to assist the family. Visits are monthly for the first 4 months and bimonthly until the year is completed. The first visit evaluates the diet made by each child and his/her family, and changes in the usual diet are proposed by making schemes, culinary recipes, example menus, etc. Most of the families were accustomed to the traditional (Mediterranean) diet, although its implementation was highly contaminated by industrial pressure. Thus, it was necessary to help them differentiate one from the other. A baseline anthropometric assessment is also performed. Patients were monitored over the course of a year, valuing weight, stature, growth, clinical evolution, treatment needs, adherence to the TMD, and the degree of satisfaction of the families. An explanatory diagram is shown in Figure 1. The study was approved by the Research Committee of the University General Hospital of Ciudad Real (Internal code: C-95, Act 03/2017).

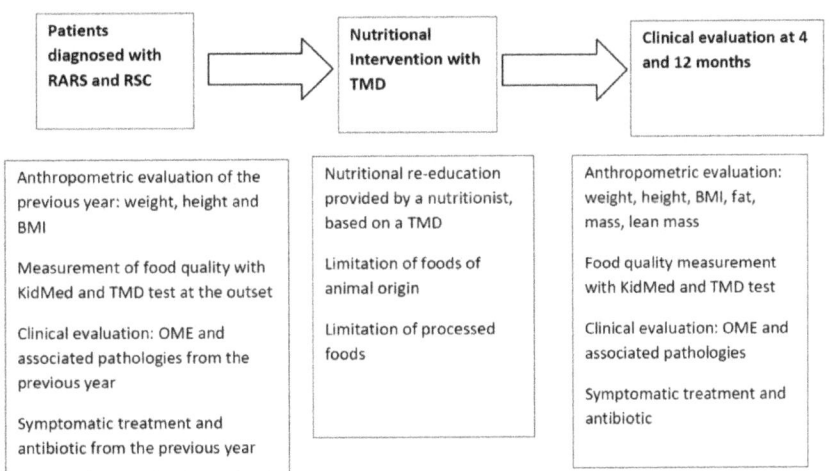

Figure 1. Study design diagram.

2.2. Study Variables: Clinical Evolution and Treatment Parameters

The study variables were the number of ARS episodes per person and year. RARS is characterized by ARS episodes that last less than 30 days and are separated from each other by at least 10 days, during which the patient is asymptomatic. The patient must present 3 ARS episodes in a period of less than 6 months, or 4 or more in a period of less than 12 months. We also took into account patients with CRS, when episodes of rhino-sinus inflammation lasted more than 90 days, with persistent residual respiratory symptoms [4,5,31].

The following variables were considered, as they are closely related to the pathology studied: upper respiratory tract infections (URTI), acute otitis media (AOM), otitis media with effusion (OME), persistent nasal obstruction (PNO), and recurrent wheezing (RW). Likewise, emergency care, symptomatic drugs, and prescribed antibiotics were assessed, all of which were assessed by person and year. A basic otorhinolaryngological examination was performed that included rhinoscopy, pharyngoscopy, otoscopy, the assessment of the presence of trans-tympanic fluid with a portable tympanometer (MicroTymp'3®, Welch Allyn, New York, NY, USA), an audiometry assessment in the collaborating children with a portable audiometer (Audioscope®, Welch Allyn, New York, NY, USA), the intentional assessment of the face (adenoid facies), a cervical lymphadenopathy, and finally a clinical assessment was made of the degree of involvement of the PNO (mild, moderate, or severe). An episode of URTI was defined by two or more of the following criteria: fever greater than 38 °C measured with a tympanic thermometer, nasal congestion or mouth breathing, runny nose, odynophagia, and cough [25]. AOM was defined following the criteria of the American Pediatric Association Guide: (1) acute presentation; (2) presence of exudate in the middle cavity of the ear demonstrated by tympanic bulging, pathological pneumatoscopy, or otorrhea; (3) inflammatory signs and symptoms such as earache or obvious redness of the eardrum [26,32]. OME was considered when the bilateral exudate or effusion persisted for more than 3 months, or more than 6 if it is unilateral [27]. PNO was defined as persistent difficulty in breathing adequately through the nose, with associated respiratory symptoms, such as mouth breathing, snoring, difficult breathing in sleep, respiratory arrest when sleeping (apnea), restless sleep, hyperflexion postures of the neck in order to sleep, drowsiness or a feeling of not having rested properly, adenoid facies, and swallowing difficulties [28]. RS or childhood asthma was defined as a situation in which three or more episodes of wheezing and/or coughing occur, in a clinical setting in which the diagnosis of asthma is the most likely, after excluding other less frequent processes [29]. In patients suspected of allergic processes, tests were carried out to rule them out.

2.3. Clinical and Therapeutic Evaluation Rate Performed on Parents or Guardians

To assess the clinical evolution of the patients, a questionnaire was designed, addressed to the parents or guardians, in which the symptoms related to RARS and CRS were evaluated, such as nasal breathing, nocturnal cough, difficulties falling asleep, recurrent colds and their complications, the intensity of the clinical symptoms, tolerance and difficulties with the diet carried out, and the degree of satisfaction with the therapeutic effects of the nutritional intervention. For each question in the questionnaire, one can answer the improvement observed with: 3: much, 2: quite, 1: something, 0: nothing. Ten questions referred to the clinic and treatment in the previous four weeks and a maximum of 30 (good control) to a minimum of 0 (poor control) was scored. A patient was considered to be poorly controlled when the total score was equal to or less than 20 (Table 1).

Table 1. Clinical and therapeutic evaluation index in rhinosinusitis. Responses from the parents or guardians regarding the improvement observed: 3: much, 2: quite, 1: something, 0: nothing.

* Average Score Obtained by All Patients	4 Months *	1 Year *
Has the number of episodes of rhinosinusitis decreased?	2.27	2.53
Have you noticed less intensity in the infectious processes?	2.67	2.93
Has the need to go to the emergency room decreased?	2.27	2.88
Have other complications decreased?	2.87	2.91
Has there been a greater recovery from the state of normality?	2.32	2.92
Have you noticed the least use of antibiotics?	2.48	2.94
Have you noticed the least use of symptomatic medications?	2.92	2.92
Has there been good diet tolerance on the part of the patient?	2.92	2.92
Has there been collaboration on dietary changes?	2.93	2.93
Are you satisfied with the results?	2.45	2.91

* is set at 4 and 12 months.

2.4. Parameters of Weight Statural Evolution

By limiting foods that are part of the new Western food culture, we have evaluated the correct weight statural development of the patients included in the study. To do this, we collected anthropometric data, such as weight, height, skinfolds, and perimeters of the arms, abdomen, and waist, and with them, we calculated the body mass index, lean mass, and body fat mass [33].

2.5. Parameters of Adherence to the TMD

To evaluate the dietary habits of patients and their families, we used the Mediterranean Diet Quality Index (KIDMED) test [34,35] and the TMD test that we presented in previous works with the intention of covering the proposed changes by the TMD [33]. The KIDMED test is one of the most prestigious for evaluating the quality of children's nutritional intake based on the TMD. It consists of a questionnaire of 16 questions that must be answered affirmatively/negatively (yes/no). Affirmative answers to the questions that represent a negative connotation in relation to the Mediterranean diet (there are four) are worth −1 point, and affirmative answers to the questions that represent a positive aspect in relation to the Mediterranean diet (there are 12) are worth +1 point. Negative answers do not score. Therefore, this index can range from 0 (minimum adherence) to 12 (maximum adherence). In order to measure the newly proposed points, we developed a complementary test (the traditional Mediterranean diet test or the TMD test) with the same structure, to which we have added nutritional and behavioral questions that—in our opinion—are not reflected in the KIDMED test. This test consists of 20 questions that must be answered affirmatively/negatively. Unlike the KIDMED test, in the TMD test, all the questions are positive. They are therefore scored with one point for each affirmative answer, and the results can range between 0 and 20 points. A test score below or equal to 7 points is considered 'poor quality', a score between 8 and 14 points is considered as 'need to improve', and scores above 15 points are considered as 'optimal traditional Mediterranean diet'. At each visit, we evaluate the nutritional tests, and together with the patients and their parents we analyze any difficulties that may have arisen and examine how we could modify the behavior to obtain the best results. Both questionnaires allow the KIDMED index and the TMD index to be calculated. According to scores obtained in the KIDMED questionnaire, three degrees of the quality of the Mediterranean diet can be obtained: (a) 'good' or 'optimal', when the score is equal to or greater than eight; (b) 'average' or 'need to improve diet or nutritional habits', when the score is between four and seven, inclusive; and (c) 'poorly adapted' or 'low-quality diet', when the score is equal to or less than three. According to the scores obtained in the TMD index, three grades are obtained: low quality ≤7, moderate quality 8–14, optimal quality >14. Physical activity and other variables of the Mediterranean lifestyle were not considered, programmed, or monitored, but rather were included only as general recommendations.

2.6. Foundations of the Traditional Mediterranean Diet

This diet is characterized by a high content of fresh, raw, perishable, and seasonal foods, rich in vegetable fiber, minerals, vitamins, enzymes, and antioxidants; an abundance of fruits, vegetables, legumes, and whole grains, one of whose characteristics is its low to moderate glycemic index; sufficient polyunsaturated fats from crude oils, nuts, seeds, and fish; low protein and saturated fat content of animal origin; and a low use of precooked and industrial foods. This means, in daily practice, the limitation of products such as white bread, industrial pastries, cow's milk, red and processed meats, sugary industrial beverages, and precooked fast food [36]. The TMD is based on the Decalogue that the Foundation of the Mediterranean diet proposes to us through its website (Table 2) [37].

Table 2. The Mediterranean diet. Ten basic recommendations.

1.	Use olive oil as your main source of added fat.
2.	Eat plenty of fruits and vegetables; fruits, vegetables, legumes, and nuts.
3.	Bread and other grain products (pasta, rice, and whole grains) should be a part of your everyday diet.
4.	Foods that have undergone minimal processing and that are fresh and locally produced are best.
5.	Consume dairy products on a daily basis, mainly yogurt and cheese.
6.	Red meat should be consumed in moderation and, if possible, as a part of stews and other recipes.
7.	Consume fish abundantly and eggs in moderation.
8.	Fresh fruit should be your everyday dessert, and sweets, cakes, and dairy desserts should be consumed only on occasion.
9.	Water is the beverage par excellence in the Mediterranean Diet.
10.	Be physically active every day since it is just as important as eating well.

This has been proclaimed a cultural heritage and an intangible heritage of humanity by Unesco [38]. In Table 3, we expose the differences between the TMD and the diet promoted by "Western civilization".

Table 3. Differences between the traditional Mediterranean diet and the "Western civilization" diet.

Traditional Mediterranean Diet	Western Civilization Diet
• Breastfeeding	• Adapted milk
• Varied, seasonal fruit	• Baby food jars and canned fruits
• Vegetables and leafy vegetables	• Baby food jars and canned vegetables and leafy vegetables
• Pulses and non-processed nuts	• Canned pulses and dried, fried, or salted nuts
• Minimally processed and fermented whole grains	• Refined, processed cereals with industrial fermenting agents
• Fermented milk, principally goat's and sheep's	• Whole, processed milks, mainly from cows
• Occasional lean meat, in small quantities	• High consumption of red, processed meats
• Minimally processed, perishable, fresh, and local foods	• Non-perishable processed and ultra-processed foods
• Limits on products with added chemicals	• Presence of chemical agents and enzyme disrupters

Sample size and statistical analysis: To calculate the sample size, a significance level of 0.05 and a power of 80% was used, assuming a decrease in the degree of involvement of ARS per patient and year of 1 unit, and a standard deviation of 3.5 units, adjusting to a 25% loss, which resulted in a sample size of 80 patients. For the analysis of the results, the statistical package SPSS 15.0 was used. A descriptive analysis was carried out with statistics of central tendency and dispersion for the quantitative variables and absolute and relative frequencies for the qualitative variables. The comparison of the results of the different variables before and after the intervention was carried out by means of the Student's t-test for paired data when the variables followed a normal distribution, or by the Wilcoxon test when they did not adjust to normal, after checking with the Shapiro–Wilk test.

3. Results

Participation was proposed in a program called 'Learning to eat from the Mediterranean'. The families of 131 patients met the RARS and RSC inclusion criteria. Nine refused to participate. From the 122 patients included, eight left the program after the first sessions. Three were due to social or personal difficulties in implementing the diet, two were due to the disagreement with the limitations of certain foods, and three were due to surgical interventions indicated by the otorhinolaryngology service and not coordinated with our team. The study was thus completed with a total of 114 patients (56 girls and 58 boys) with an average age of 2.9 years. All of the patients included in the study were evaluated at 4 and 12 months after the initial visit. The results obtained were similar in both sexes, and are thus collated together (Table 4).

Table 4. Sample characteristics. The average age is 2.6 years.

	Boys (n = 56) *	Girls (n = 58) *
Weight (kg)	14.93 ± 3.35	13.91 ± 3.21
Height (m)	0.94 ± 0.10	0.93 ± 0.11
BMI (kg/m^2)	16.47 ± 1.36	15.80 ± 1.29
Fat mass (%)	14.94 ± 2.67	14.90 ± 2.05
Lean mass (%)	12.61 ± 2.78	11.77 ± 2.37

* Mean ± standard deviation; BMI: body mass index.

Table 5 shows the evolution of the patients with the number of ARS episodes in the previous year and the following year after the application of the nutritional program; ARS episodes per child and year were assessed. The evolution of other bacterial complications of the oropharynx is also exposed.

Table 5. Evolution during the previous year and during the year of treatment.

	Previous Year *	Year of Treatment *	p
Number of episodes of acute rhinosinusitis (ARS) per child and year	3.37 ± 1.21	0.32 ± 0.47	0.01
Number of upper respiratory tract infections (URTI) per child and year	7.31 ± 1.43	2.79 ± 0.67	0.01
Degree of involvement of persistent nasal obstruction (PNO): 0 (mild); 1 (moderate); 2 (intense).	1.89 ± 0.30	0.06 ± 0.08	0.03
Others bacterial complications of the oropharynx, by child and year	4.31 ± 0.25	0.72 ± 0.31	0.02
Emergencies per child and year	2.17 ± 0.75	0.25 ± 0.14	0.03
Antibiotics treatment cycles per child and year	3.71 ± 0.67	0.46 ± 0.28	0.01
Number of symptomatic treatment per child and year	6.82 ± 1.26	2.94 ± 0.89	0.02

* Mean ± standard deviation.

We have evaluated the degree of clinical involvement of children with RARS and CRS and we have recorded the mean of their total score before and after the treatment. We have also assessed the number of times the patients visited the emergency department in the previous year and the following year, as well as the antibiotic treatment cycles they received during their inflammatory processes and symptomatic treatment, such as paracetamol, saline sprays, anti-inflammatory drugs, or expectorant mucolytics (Figure 2).

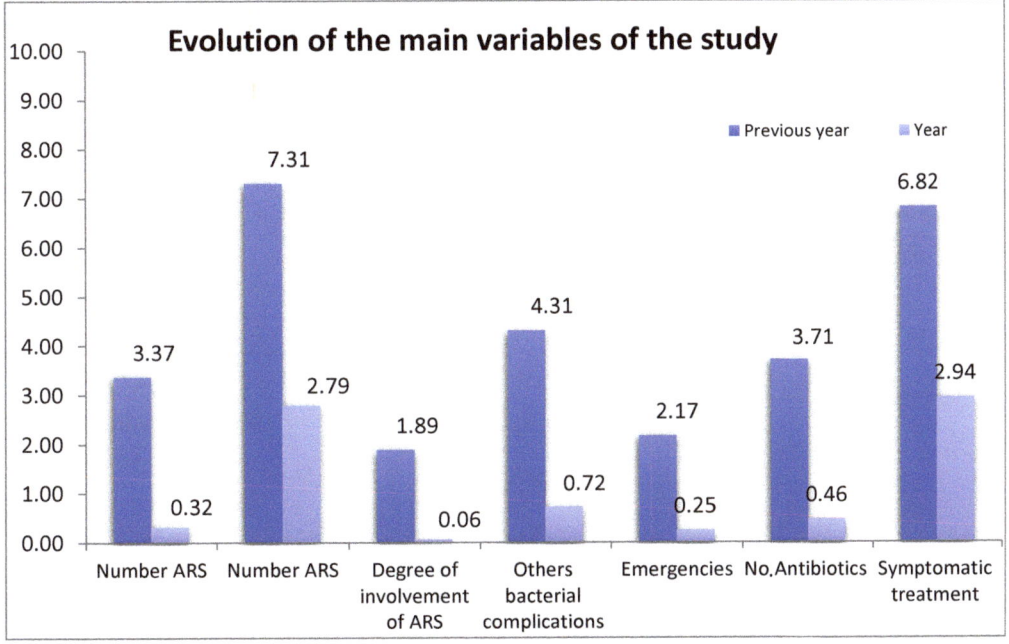

Figure 2. Evolution of the main variables of the study.

The clinical evaluation test of the patients is shown in Table 1, which shows the assessment of the families regarding the evolution of the process and the difficulties of treatment. The anthropometric variables before, at four months, and after intervention, are set out in Table 6. The mean weight increase the year before the study was 2.33 kg compared to the current 2.64 kg, and the increase in average height was 8.8 cm compared to 9.4 cm today.

Table 6. Anthropometric assessment at the start, after four months, and after one year.

	At the Start of Treatment *	4 Months of Treatment *	1 Year of Treatment *	p
BMI (body mass index)	16.13 ± 1.42	15.91 ± 1.23	15.80 ± 1.38	0.02
Fat mass (%)	14.91 ± 2.72	14.72 ± 2.55	14.80 ± 2.39	0.02
Lean mass (%)	12.19 ± 2.49	13.00 ± 2.28	14.44 ± 2.18	0.03

* Mean ± standard deviation.

The mean value of the KIDMED index at the beginning of the program was 7.7 ± 1.82 points; 24.6% of the patients obtained a qualification according to the KIDMED test of "need to improve" and 69.3% obtained the qualification of "optimal diet". At the end of the study, 90.4% of the children obtained optimal levels with a mean of 11 points, mean difference of 2.11 ± 0.10 (95% CI: 1.91–2.31 $p < 0.01$). According to this data, the average value of the KIDMED index evolved from a score considered medium-high at the beginning of the program to an optimal value at the end of the program (Table 7, Figures 3 and 4).

Table 7. The KIDMED test (%).

	At the Start	After 4 Months	After 1 Year
One piece of fruit per day	75.4	66.2	85.1
One+ piece of fruit per day	20.2	17.7	78.9
One vegetable per day	71.9	63.1	84.2
Vegetables more than once per day	10.5	9.2	63.2
Regularly eats fresh fish (2–3 times/week)	76.3	66.9	84.2
Visits fast food restaurant once or more per week	17.5	15.4	0.9
Legumes 1–2 times/week	78.9	69.3	85.1
Pasta and rice every week	78.1	68.5	84.2
Cereal or derivative for breakfast	81.6	71.6	84.2
Regularly eats dried fruit and nuts	14.9	13.1	42.1
Olive oil used at home	82.5	72.3	85.1
No breakfast	10.5	9.2	4.4
Dairy at breakfast	82.5	72.3	84.2
Factory-baked goods for breakfast	33.3	29.2	0.9
Two yoghurts or 40 g cheese/day	78.1	68.5	84.2
Sweets and snacks every day	27.2	23.9	4.4

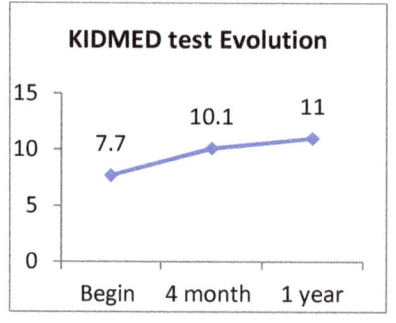 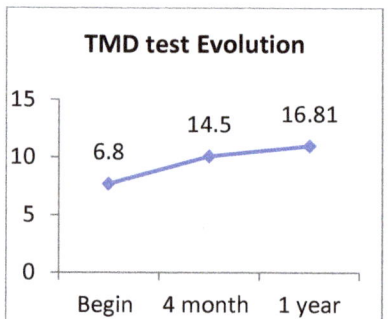

Figure 3. The KIDMED and the TMD tests evolution.

At the beginning of the study, the mean value of the TMD test was 6.79 ± 1.98, qualifying as a poor-quality diet; 89.5% of the sample obtained a score below eight points (poor-quality diet) and 10.5% obtained a score between eight and fourteen points (need for improvement). At the end of the study, the mean score was 16.78 ± 1.90 points, qualifying as an optimal traditional Mediterranean diet. The TMD test evolved from levels considered to be low quality to optimal levels (Table 8 and Figure 5). Despite the good score obtained with the KIDMED test, the patients maintained the incidence of ARS. However, when applying the TMD test, we obtained statistically significant results in the evolution of ARS.

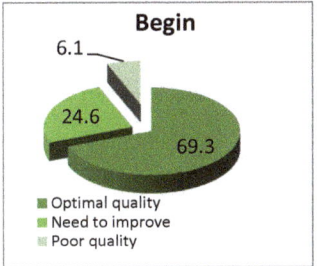 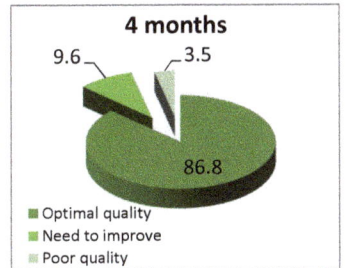 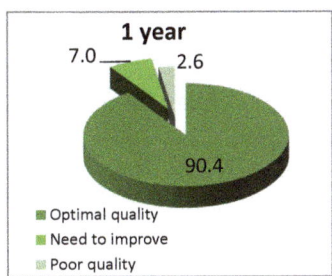

Figure 4. Evolution of the quality of diet, measured using the KIDMED test.

Table 8. The traditional Mediterranean diet test (%).

	Start	4 Months	Year
Minimum two pieces of fruit every day.	28.9	76.3	92.1
Fresh vegetables at every meal, as a first course, or as part of the main course	32.5	58.8	71.9
Limited sugar intake (sweetened breakfast cereal, sweetened yoghurts or milkshakes, cakes, soft drinks, sugary biscuits, sweets, ice-cream, etc.).	12.3	72.8	80.7
Sporadic use of potatoes (1–2 times/week) and preferably not fried.	26.3	77.2	86.0
Enjoys legumes and eats them one or more times a week, not always accompanied by meat.	23.7	69.3	79.8
Regular intake of white fish, oily fish, and seafood (2–3 times/week).	73.7	77.2	88.6
Consumes whole grains (whole wheat pasta, brown rice, whole wheat bread, etc.) in a controlled way, and limits the consumption of refined flour, such as white bread, to less than 40g per day.	14.0	72.8	83.3
Limit the consumption of preservatives and hydrogenated vegetable fats, regularly using unprocessed homemade foods.	21.9	64.9	83.3
Dairy: ingested, preferably skimmed in the form of natural yogurt, and preferably goat or sheep cheese, avoiding the use of sugary yogurts, dairy desserts, creams, margarines, ice creams, etc.	13.2	66.7	80.7
Only lean processed meats, less than twice per week.	14.9	70.2	85.1
Preferably white meat, less than three times per week (lean).	24.6	77.2	73.7
30–50% of your daily menu consists of raw or undercooked foods (fruits, vegetables, greens, soups, purees, raw nuts, extra virgin olive oil, etc.), preferably choosing seasonal ones.	6.1	36.0	56.1
Junk food (indoors or outdoors) no more than one time per week.	37.7	78.9	80.7
Consumes, as main fats, extra virgin olive oil and raw nuts. Avoids poor quality industrial greases.	39.5	80.7	85.1
Has a quality breakfast or lunch.	35.1	60.5	84.2
Does not peck between meals.	23.7	58.8	88.6
Adapts to the food made at home (family) and alternatives not offered.	28.9	46.5	87.7
Mealtimes together, avoiding the television or other technology.	57.9	80.7	82.5
Regular physical exercise (running, playing, walking, climbing, etc.) or sport.	73.7	76.3	81.6
Gets 7–9 h of sleep daily.	68.1	85.1	89.2

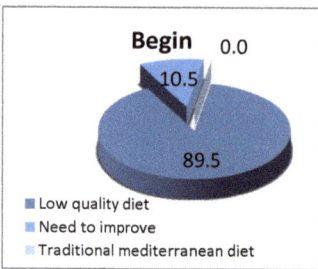 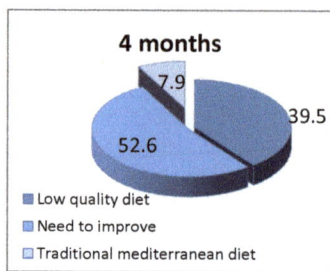 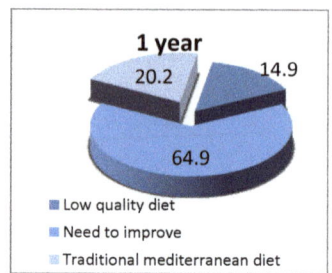

Figure 5. Evolution of the quality of diet, measured using the TMD test.

4. Discussion

In view of these results, we suggest that the traditional Mediterranean diet could help in the prevention and also in the control of RARS and CRS, improve their treatment, and limit pharmacological and surgical intervention. At the end of the year of the intervention, less than 5% of the patients treated met the criteria to be classified as having RARS and CRS. Of the patients, 53.5% did not have any ARS, and 26.3% had only one, when the usual issue with the conventional treatment is that new episodes would have been repeated and would have ended up in the OR service. We had few episodes of CRS, probably because many of the patients already followed an acceptable Mediterranean diet, and because when they reached three to four annual episodes of ARS, we incorporated them into the TMD. RARS and CRS often overlap and it is difficult to know when a new rhinosinusitis episode starts or when it is a relapse of a process that has not yet been resolved [5]. In our study, most of the patients were diagnosed with RARS.

The number of ARS episodes decreased by 90.5%, from a mean of 3.37 to less than 0.32% episodes per year. Although with age the effectiveness of the immune system increases and recurrent inflammatory episodes tend to disappear spontaneously, such a rapid evolution in the disappearance of symptoms could not be anticipated, which resulted in preventing the patients from having prolonged pharmacological treatments and undergoing surgery. Thus, we deduce that the nutritional intervention was beneficial for them. The degree of intensity of the ARS decreased significantly, so that not only did the total number of ARS episodes decrease, but there was also less involvement and fewer symptoms in the patients who followed the nutritional guidelines. It is important to note that during the time that the patients were enrolled in the study, we were extending the application of the TMD to the entire pediatric population (siblings, relatives, patients with other recurrent pathologies, and infants under two years of age). This led to a progressive decrease in the number of patients diagnosed with ARS, thus delaying the achievement of the sample size [30]. As we had already verified in previous studies, the URTI [25], which are one of the precipitating reasons for bacterial involvement of the paranasal sinuses, decreased significantly. In our study, there was 60% less URTI than in the previous year.

The number of other bacterial complications decreased by 88.8% (4.31 in the previous year versus 0.72 in the year of intervention); 61% of the patients did not have any bacterial complication during the nutritional intervention period, 28% had only one in the entire year, and 10% had two, compared to the more than four episodes they had on average in the previous year. Children with PNO went from a mild-moderate intensity profile to not at all-mild [28]. Likewise, one of the most frequent reasons for attending pediatric emergencies is the discomfort caused by ARS, with worsening of the URTI and difficulties in breathing through the nose and being able to fall asleep; there was a significant reduction of 88.5% in emergencies compared to the previous year. As a consequence of the decrease in URTI, ARS, and other bacterial complications, symptomatic treatment decreased by 57%. Likewise, antibiotic treatment was reduced by 87.6%, which allows us to verify a greater benignity of the infectious processes. The degree of satisfaction shown by the parents in the clinical evaluation test was high, with scores indicating a good clinical and therapeutic evolution. In the first four months, improvements were already observed compared to the situation of the previous year, so that loyalty increased and monitoring was easier.

There was a good tolerance to the proposed diet, with easy adaptation and without great culinary difficulties. The main difficulty was the fulfillment of the diet, as they were proposed to make a homemade, familiar diet of fresh products that must be prepared, and the parents did not always have the time and dedication to do it properly. The presence of a dietitian-nutritionist was essential to guarantee the compliance with the the TMD. By the end of the program, the dietary habits of the patients had improved in the sample as a whole; an increase in the number of patients consuming fruits, vegetables, nuts, whole grains, and fermented dairy products was observed. In general, the consumption of proteins of animal origin was reduced considerably, especially cow's milk, red meat, and meat products. The consumption of processed foods also decreased, especially industrial pastries. Prior to the development of our study, we promoted the application of a validated test, such as the KIDMED test [34], with the intention of preventing and treating inflammatory and recurrent diseases, as well as preventing becoming overweight and obese [33]. Despite this, we did not obtain satisfactory results, so we decided to implement a new TMD test, which collected information about important aspects of the Mediterranean diet that had not previously been detailed. Many of the children who had an optimal KIDMED test failed on the TMD index. It was only when they began to show improved scores with the new test that we obtained satisfactory results. In the KIDMED test, some variables that we believe are important are not considered. For example, no differences are noted between refined cereals and whole grains, nor are there any references to the consumption of sugar or sugary industrial juices. Additionally, in general, glycemic index/glycemic load is not taken into account. In the lipid section, saturated fat consumption is neither limited nor evaluated. The test does not allow for the detection of an excess consumption of animal proteins. Additionally, no assessment is made of the consumption of raw food, nor is the minimum amount to be taken specified. Serving sizes and schedules are not taken into account. Completing the KIDMED test has not been shown to be effective in our study. We believe that these small nuances that we have proposed in the TMD test are important for obtaining satisfactory results in the examination of recurrent inflammatory diseases, in particular RARS. The patients showed satisfactory predicted growth rates. Their weight, height, and BMI percentile evolved as expected. A positive result was the slight decrease in the BMI and fat mass levels and a small increase in height and lean body mass.

Although these data suggest that the intake of healthy foods and/or the avoidance of non-traditional foods may play an important role in the control of ARS, there are almost no bibliographic references in the scientific literature. We want to highlight that most of the studies published on the treatment of RARS and CRS are based on the application of actions external to the body, such as the use of drugs or surgical intervention. The nutritional factors have not been taken into account, when the deconfiguration of the inflammatory system and the immune system due to inadequate food is likely at the base of these pathologies. The etiology and pathogenesis of this inflammation are often unclear, although this is believed to represent an inappropriate or excessive immune response to an external stimulus inhaled through the nasal airways [1].

The research has suggested the protective effect of breastfeeding for at least 6 months, although other risk factors accumulate after that age [39]. Among them, the early introduction of adapted milk has been noted [40] as well as the abuse of antibiotics [41]. A pan-European study has shown that children consuming excessive refined flours and processed animal-based products and having a diet poor in fruit and vegetables have high inflammatory markers, and as a whole, they can be considered to be in a pro-inflammatory state [42]. Likewise, ARS patients have been shown to have an altered regulation of key immune mediators during good health and pathogenesis and are amenable to treatment by immunomodulatory intervention [43]. Predominantly eating foods with a low glycemic index/load—typical of the TMD—helps to control insulin levels; this hormone may interfere in the formation of anti-inflammatory eicosanoids, by blocking the Δ-desaturase enzyme [44].

Similarly, the TMD is rich in vitamins, minerals, and antioxidants, many of which are indispensable co-factors in the enzymatic chemical reactions involved in the body's immune processes. Children with recurrent inflammatory infections have been shown to have poor responses to pro-inflammatory cytokines and antiviral chemokines [45,46]. High-mobility group box protein 1 (HMGB1), that acts as a mediator between innate and acquired immunity, is overexpressed and can play a role in the progression of CRS and RARS, acting as an inflammatory marker and cytokine [47].

There is a growing interest in understanding the alterations of the naso-sinus microbiome as a causative factor of the disease. Likewise, it has been considered that there is a dysfunctional naso-sinus mucosa, in which defects of the epithelial surface may be the basis of the etiology and pathogenesis of the disorder [48–51]. It has been shown that an inadequate diet, away from the traditional diet, can alter the rhino-sinus microbiota and cause intestinal dysbiosis [52]. Biofilms provide a protected environment for pathogens and can be responsible for persistent or recurrent diseases [1]. The immune system may not recognize foreign, infrequent, or foreign microbial germs, and cause the cytokines or other cell signaling molecules to react, which alter inflammatory mechanisms and leave the respiratory mucosa in a permanent pro-inflammatory state. In this way, in the face of small stimuli, such as simple catarrhal viruses, hyper-reactivity of the mucous membranes would be triggered, with flowery symptoms, which would end up causing the usual complications and in particular the RARS. Adenoid hypertrophy and adenoiditis contribute significantly to the pathogenesis of RARS, being one of the main differences between the involvement of children and adults [1,53]. The mechanisms by which the intestinal flora modulates the immune response are not clear, but it seems prudent to favor an intestinal microbiota typical of the human species, since evolution and genetic coding have had to configure a specific symbiosis between nutrition, the intestinal microbiota, and immunity that we should not modify.

The growing interest in the Mediterranean diet is based on its role in inflammatory diseases [54]. Several clinical and epidemiological studies, as well as experimental studies, show that the consumption of the TMD reduces the incidence of certain pathologies related to oxidative stress, chronic inflammation, and the immune system, such as cancer, atherosclerosis, or cardiovascular disease [55]. There is evidence that diet and individual nutrients can influence the systemic markers of immune function and inflammation [56]. The pro-inflammatory actions of platelet-activating factor (PAF), one of the most potent endogenous mediators of inflammation, can be favorably modulated by the TMD and regulate its metabolism [57]. The TMD is an ancient diet, dating back to way before documented history, and which has stood the test of time. Many of the foodstuffs eaten as part of the Western diet contain materials not recognized or assimilated by the human body. Many of these products are not absorbed by the intestine, thus encouraging non-specific microflora that is alien to the human intestinal microbiota. The excess "antigenic load" inherent in the Western diet of today—which has multiplied the available foodstuffs by the thousand—may misadjust our immune system, making it weaker and notably hyperplasic.

It has recently been proven that better adherence to the Mediterranean diet may be associated with a lower risk of COVID-19 [58,59], demonstrating its effect against virus infections. Secretory IgA antibodies are an important part of the immune defense against viral diseases. People who ingest Okinawan vegetables have high IgA levels and might be more likely to develop immunity against influenza RNA viruses [60].

One of the characteristics that every research study should have is that it is easily reproducible, using small groups, and with little economic cost. The work presented here is easy to reproduce in any primary care pediatric consultation, but it is not easy to perform due to the lack of nutritionists and the lack of effective monitoring of the diet.

We could not perform a study with a control group since most of our pediatric space was adhering to the Mediterranean diet and it did not seem ethical to promote a pro-inflammatory Western-type diet in a control group. Our hypothesis is precisely that the standard diet proposed by "Western civilization" is the origin of alterations in the inflammatory and immune mechanisms, and therefore the precipitating factor of most of the inflammatory and recurrent diseases of childhood. It would have been very interesting to perform analyses that measured the response of the immune system, inflammatory markers, and the data on the modification of the microbiota when making the nutritional change.

Most of our patients have been consecutively included in the program "Learning to eat from the Mediterranean" and we have verified how the prevalence of ARS and other inflammatory recurrent diseases has decreased considerably. The change of the "model of medicine" that these research studies entail should not go unnoticed. It is no longer about remedying a disease with external drugs or surgical interventions, but the therapeutic proposal is based on providing the body with everything it needs to solve their needs and eliminate that for which it is not ready.

We can conclude by saying that the application of the traditional Mediterranean diet could have promising effects in the prevention and treatment of acute recurrent and chronic rhinosinusitis, with a notable decrease in associated inflammatory diseases, limiting pharmacological and surgical intervention in many of these patients.

Author Contributions: Conceptualization, F.M.C.-S.; and B.C.; methodology, F.M.C.-S.; software, B.C.; validation, F.M.C.-S.; B.C., and A.C.; formal analysis, B.C.; investigation, F.M.C.-S.; B.C., and A.C.; re-sources, F.M.C.-S.; data curation, B.C.; writing—original draft preparation, F.M.C.-S.; writing—review and editing, F.M.C.-S.; visualization, F.M.C.-S. All authors have read and agreed to the published version of the manuscript.

Funding: This research received no external funding.

Institutional Review Board Statement: The study was conducted according to the guidelines of the Declaration of Helsinki, and approved by the Institutional Review Board (or Ethics Committee) of Hospital General Universitario de Ciudad Real (Internal code: C-95, Act 03/2017).

Informed Consent Statement: Informed consent was obtained from all subjects involved in the study.

Conflicts of Interest: The authors declare no conflict of interest.

References

1. Quintanilla-Dieck, L.; Lam, D.J. Chronic Rhinosinusitis in Children. *Curr. Treat. Options Pediatr.* **2018**, *4*, 413–424. [CrossRef]
2. Gilani, S.; Shin, J.J. The Burden and Visit Prevalence of Pediatric Chronic Rhinosinusitis. *Otolaryngol. Neck Surg.* **2017**, *157*, 1048–1052. [CrossRef]
3. Brietzke, S.E.; Shin, J.J.; Choi, S.; Lee, J.T.; Parikh, S.R.; Pena, M.; Prager, J.D.; Ramadan, H.; Veling, M.; Corrigan, M.; et al. Clinical Consensus Statement. *Otolaryngol. Neck Surg.* **2014**, *151*, 542–553. [CrossRef]
4. Martínez, L.; Albañil, R.; De la Flor, J.; Piñeiro RCervera, J.; Baquero Artigao, F.; Alfayate Miguelez, S.; Moraga Llop, F.; Cilleruelo Ortega, M.J.; Calvo Rey, C. Consensus document on the aetiology, diagnosis and treatment of sinusitis. *An. Pediatr.* **2013**, *79*, 330.e1–330.e12.
5. Orlandi, R.R.; Kingdom, T.T.; Hwang, P.H.; Smith, T.L.; Alt, J.A.; Baroody, F.M.; Batra, P.S.; Bernal-Sprekelsen, M.; Bhattacharyya, N.; Chandra, R.K.; et al. International Consensus Statement on Allergy and Rhinology: Rhinosinusitis. *Int. Forum Allergy Rhinol.* **2016**, *6*, S22–S209. [CrossRef]
6. Gallant, J.-N.; Basem, J.; Turner, J.; Shannon, C.N.; Virgin, F.W. Nasal saline irrigation in pediatric rhinosinusitis: A systematic review. *Int. J. Pediatr. Otorhinolaryngol.* **2018**, *108*, 155–162. [CrossRef]
7. Fokkens, W.J.; Lund, V.J.; Mullol, J.; Bachert, C.; Alobid, I.; Baroody, F.; Cohen, N.; Cervin, A.; Douglas, R.; Gevaert, P.; et al. European position paper on rhinosinusitis and nasal polyps. *Rhinology* **2012**, *50*, 1–12. [CrossRef] [PubMed]
8. Chandy, Z.; Ference, E.; Lee, J.T. Clinical guidelines on chronic rhinosinusitis in children. *Curr. Allergy Asthma Rep.* **2019**, *19*, 14. [CrossRef] [PubMed]
9. Wald, E.R.; Applegate, K.; Bordley, C.; Darrow, D.H.; Glode, M.P.; Marcy, S.M.; E Nelson, C.; Rosenfeld, R.M.; Shaikh, N.; Smith, M.J.; et al. Clinical Practice Guideline for the Diagnosis and Management of Acute Bacterial Sinusitis in Children Aged 1 to 18 Years. *Pediatrics* **2013**, *132*, e262–e280. [CrossRef] [PubMed]
10. Licari, A.; Brambilla, I.; Castagnoli, R.; Marseglia, A.; Paganelli, V.; Foiadelli, T.; Marseglia, G.L. Rhinosinutis and Asthma in Children. *Sinusitis* **2018**, *3*, 3. [CrossRef]
11. Ebell, M.H.; McKay, B.; Guilbault, R.; Ermias, Y. Diagnosis of acute rhinosinusitis in primary care: A systematic review of test accuracy. *Br. J. Gen. Pract.* **2016**, *66*, e612–e632. [CrossRef] [PubMed]

12. Shapiro, D.J.; Gonzales, R.; Cabana, M.D.; Hersh, A.l. National trends in visit rates and antibiotic prescribing for children whit acute sinusitis. *Pediatrics* **2011**, *127*, 28–34. [CrossRef] [PubMed]
13. Hopp, R.J. Pediatric Chronic Rhinosinusitis: Unmet Needs. *Sinusitis* **2020**, *4*, 2–7. [CrossRef]
14. Hopp, R.; Allison, J.; Brooks, D. Fifty Years of Chronic Rhinosinusitis in Children: The Accepted, the Unknown, and Thoughts for the Future. *Pediatr. Allergy Immunol. Pulmonol.* **2016**, *29*, 61–67. [CrossRef]
15. Callén Blecua, M.; Garmendia Iglesias, M.A. Sinusitis. The Pediatrician of Care Primary and Sinusitis Protocols of the GVR (Publication P-GVR-7). Available online: https://www.respirar.org/images/sinusitis-2013.pdf (accessed on 22 June 2021).
16. Hopp, R.J. Diagnosis and manging chronic pediatric rhinosinusitis: Still more questions than answers. *Arch. Immunol. Allergy* **2019**, *2*, 35–41.
17. Head, K.; Chong, L.Y.; Piromchai, P.; Hopkins, C.; Philpott, C.; Schilder, A.G.; Burton, M.J. Systemic and topical antibiotics for chronic rhinosinusitis. *Cochrane Database Syst. Rev.* **2016**, *4*. [CrossRef] [PubMed]
18. Chong, L.Y.; Head, K.; Hopkins, C.; Philpott, C.; Schilder, A.G.M.; Burton, M.J. Intranasal steroids versus placebo or no intervention for chronic rhinosinusitis. *Cochrane Database Syst. Rev.* **2016**, *4*, CD011996. [CrossRef]
19. Head, K.; Chong, L.Y.; Hopkins, C.; Philpott, C.; Burton, M.J.; Schilldler, A.G. Short-course oral steroids alone for chronic rhinosinusitis. *Cochrane Database Syst Rev.* **2016**. [CrossRef]
20. Duse, M.; Santamaria, F.; Verga, M.C.; Bergamini, M.; Simeone, G.; Leonardi, L.; Tezza, G.; Bianchi, A.; Capuano, A.; Cardinale, F.; et al. Inter-society consensus for the use of inhaled corticosteroids in infants, children and adolescents with airway diseases. *Ital. J. Pediatr.* **2021**, *47*, 97. [CrossRef] [PubMed]
21. Shaikh, N.; Wald, E.R. Decongestants, antihistamines and nasal irrigation for acute sinusitis in children. *Cochrane Database Syst. Rev.* **2014**, *2014*, CD007909. [CrossRef]
22. Runkle, K. Decongestants, antihistamines and nasal irrigation for acute sinusitis in children. *Paediatr. Child Health* **2016**, *21*, 143–144. [CrossRef] [PubMed]
23. Beswick, D.M.; Messner, A.H.; Hwang, P.H. Pediatric Chronic Rhinosinusitis Management in Rhinologists and Pediatric Otolaryngologists. *Ann. Otol. Rhinol. Laryngol.* **2017**, *126*, 634–639. [CrossRef] [PubMed]
24. Kargın, D.; Tomaino, L.; Serra-Majem, L. Experimental Outcomes of the Mediterranean Diet: Lessons Learned from the Predimed Randomized Controlled Trial. *Nutrients* **2019**, *11*, 2991. [CrossRef] [PubMed]
25. Calatayud, F.; Calatayud, B.; Gallego, J.; González-Martín, C.; Alguacil, L. Effects of Mediterranean diet in patients with recurring colds and frequent complications. *Allergol. Immunopathol.* **2017**, *45*, 417–424. [CrossRef] [PubMed]
26. Calatayud-Sáez, F.M.; Calatayud, B.; Calatayud, A. Recurrent acute otitis media could be related to the pro-inflammatory state that causes an incorrect diet. *Prog. Nutr.*. Pending publication.
27. Calatayud-Sáez, F.; Calatayud, B.; Calatayud, A. Effects of the Traditional Mediterranean Diet in Patients with Otitis Media with Effusion. *Nutrients* **2021**, *13*, 2181. [CrossRef]
28. Calatayud-Sáez, F.; Calatayud, B.; Calatayud, A. Persistent Nasal Obstruction: An Expression of the Pro-Inflammatory State? *Sinusitis* **2021**, *5*, 90–100. [CrossRef]
29. Calatayud-Sáez, F.M.; del Prado, B.C.M.; Fernández-Pacheco, J.G.; González-Martín, C.; Merino, L.A. Mediterranean diet and childhood asthma. *Allergol. Immunopathol.* **2016**, *44*, 99–105. [CrossRef]
30. Calatayud-Sáez, F.M.; Calatayud, B.; Luque, M.; Calatayud, A.; Gallego, J.G.; Rivas, F. Effects of affinity to the Mediterranean Diet pattern along with breastfeeding on childhood asthma, inflammatory and recurrent diseases in an intervention study. *Authorea* **2020**. Preprint, pending review. [CrossRef]
31. Callén, M.; Garmendia, M.A. Sinusitis. The Primary Care Pediatrician and Sinusitis GVR Protocols. *(publication P-GVR-7)*. Available online: https://www.respirar.org/images/sinusitis-2013.pdf (accessed on 26 June 2021).
32. American Academy of Pediatrics and American Academy of Family Physicians. Diagnosis and management of acute otitis media. *Pediatrics* **2004**, *113*, 1451–1465. [CrossRef]
33. Calatayud-Sáez, F.M.; Calatayud, B. Efficacy of the recommendation of a Mediterranean diet pattern in preschoolers with overweight and obesity. *Acta Pediátr. Esp.* **2020**, *78*, e101–e110.
34. Serra, L.; Ribas, L.; Ngo, J.; Ortega, R.M.; Pérez, C.; Aranceta, J. Food, youth and the Mediterranean diet in Spain. Development of the KIDMED, quality index of the Mediterranean diet in childhood and adolescence. In *Infant and Youth Nutrition. I Study enKid*. Barcelona: Masson; Serra, L., Aranceta, J., Eds.; 2002; Available online: https://www.casadellibro.com/libro-alimentacion-infantil-y-juvenil-estudio-enkid/9788445812549/856399 (accessed on 28 June 2021).
35. Serra, L.; Ribas, L.; Aranceta, J.; Pérez, C.; Saavedra, P.; Peña, L. Childhood and youth obesity in Spain. *EnKid study results (1998–2000) Med. Clin.* **2003**, *121*, 725–732.
36. Márquez-Sandoval, F.; Bulló, M.; Vizmanos, B.; Casas-Agustench, P.; Salas-Salvadó, J. A healthy eating pattern: The traditional Mediterranean diet. *Antropo* **2008**, *16*, 11–22.
37. Foundation of the Mediterranean Diet. 10 Basic Recommendations of the Mediterranean Diet. Available online: http://fdmed.org/dieta-mediterranea/decalogo/ (accessed on 28 June 2021).
38. WHO. *Overweight and Obesity*; World Health Organization: Geneva, Switzerland, 2006; Available online: https://ich.unesco.org/en/RL/mediterranean-diet-00884?RL=00884 (accessed on 28 June 2021).

39. Brennan-Jones, C.G.; Eikelboom, R.H.; Jacques, A.; Swanepoel, D.W.; Atlas, M.D.; Whitehouse, A.J.; Jamieson, S.E.; Oddy, W.H. Protective benefit of predominant breastfeeding against otitis media may be limited to early childhood: Results from a prospective birth cohort study. *Clin. Otolaryngol.* **2016**, *42*, 29–37. [CrossRef] [PubMed]
40. Chonmaitree, T.; Trujillo, R.; Jennings, K.; Alvarez-Fernandez, P.; Patel, J.A.; Loeffelholz, M.J.; Nokso-Koivisto, J.; Matalon, R.; Pyles, R.B.; Miller, A.L.; et al. Acute Otitis Media and Other Complications of Viral Respiratory Infection. *Pediatrics* **2016**, *137*, e20153555. [CrossRef]
41. Bezáková, N.; Damoiseaux, R.A.; Hoes, A.W.; Schilder, A.G.; Rovers, M.M. Recurrence up to 3.5 years after antibiotic treatment of acute otitis media in very young Dutch children: Survey of trial participants. *BMJ* **2009**, *338*, b2525. [CrossRef]
42. González-Gil, E.M.; Tognon, G.; Lissner, L.; Intemann, T.; Pala, V.; Galli, C.; Wolters, M.; Siani, A.; Veidebaum, T.; Michels, N.; et al. Prospective associations between dietary patterns and high sensitivity C-reactive protein in European children: The IDEFICS study. *Eur. J. Nutr.* **2018**, *57*, 1397–1407. [CrossRef]
43. Yaqoob, P. Mechanisms underlying the immunomodulatory effects of n-3 PUFA. *Proc. Nutr. Soc.* **2010**, *69*, 311–315. [CrossRef]
44. Gil, A.; Sánchez de Medina, F. Intercellular communication: Hormones, eicosanoides and cytokines. Capit. 3 of de Treaty of Nutrition, Gil A. Volume I. Physiological and biochmical bases of nutrition. Ed. Panamericana. 2010.
45. Ren, D.; Xu, Q.; Almudevar, A.L.; E Pichichero, M. Impaired Proinflammatory Response in Stringently Defined Otitis-prone Children During Viral Upper Respiratory Infections. *Clin. Infect. Dis.* **2018**, *68*, 1566–1574. [CrossRef]
46. Guilleminault, L.; Williams, E.J.; Scott, H.A.; Berthon, B.S.; Jensen, M.; Wood, L.G. Diet and Asthma: Is It Time to Adapt Our Message? *Nutrients* **2017**, *9*, 1227. [CrossRef]
47. Ciprandi, G.; Bellussi, L.M.; Passali, G.C.; Damiani, V.; Passali, D. HMGB1 in nasal inflammatory diseases: A reappraisal 30 years after its discovery. *Expert Rev. Clin. Immunol.* **2020**, *16*, 457–463. [CrossRef] [PubMed]
48. Hopp, R.J. Pediatric Chronic Sinusitis: What are thou? A Clinical Opinion. *Sinusitis* **2017**, *2*, 6. [CrossRef]
49. Silviu-Dan, F.; Fanny, S.D. Pediatric Chronic Rhinosinusitis. *Pediatr. Ann.* **2014**, *43*, 201–209. [CrossRef] [PubMed]
50. Bose, S.; Grammer, L.C.; Peters, A.T. Infectious Chronic Rhinosinusitis. *J. Allergy Clin. Immunol. Pract.* **2016**, *4*, 584–589. [CrossRef]
51. Pasha, M.A. State-of-the-Art Adult Chronic Rhinosinusitis Microbiome: Perspective for Future Studies in Pediatrics. *Sinusitis* **2018**, *3*, 1. [CrossRef]
52. Hamilos, D.L. Pediatric Chronic Rhinosinusitis. *Am. J. Rhinol. Allergy* **2015**, *29*, 414–420. [CrossRef] [PubMed]
53. Rojas, V.; Ruz, P.; Valdés, C. Chronic rhinosinusitis in children: Review of the evaluation and current management. *Rev. Otorrinolaringol. Cir. Cabeza Cuello* **2020**, *80*, 237–246, ISSN 0718-4816. [CrossRef]
54. Tsigalou, C.; Konstantinidis, T.; Paraschaki, A.; Stavropoulou, E.; Voidarou, C.; Bezirtzoglou, E. Mediterranean Diet as a Tool to Combat Inflammation and Chronic Diseases. An Overview. *Biomedicines* **2020**, *8*, 201. [CrossRef]
55. Casas, R.; Estruch, R.; Sacanella, E. The Protective Effects of Extra Virgin Olive Oil on Immune-mediated Inflammatory Responses. *Endocr. Metab. Immune Disord.-Drug Targets* **2017**, *18*, 23–35. [CrossRef]
56. Venter, C.; Eyerich, S.; Sarin, T.; Klatt, K.C. Nutrition and the Immune System: A Complicated Tango. *Nutrients* **2020**, *12*, 818. [CrossRef]
57. Nomikos, T.; Fragopoulou, E.; Antonopoulou, S.; Panagiotakos, D.B. Mediterranean diet and platelet-activating factor; a systematic review. *Clin. Biochem.* **2018**, *60*, 1–10. [CrossRef] [PubMed]
58. Perez-Araluce, R.; Martinez-Gonzalez, M.; Fernández-Lázaro, C.; Bes-Rastrollo, M.; Gea, A.; Carlos, S. Mediterranean diet and the risk of COVID-19 in the 'Seguimiento Universidad de Navarra' cohort. *Clin. Nutr.* **2021**, *15*. in Press. [CrossRef]
59. Iddir, M.; Brito, A.; Dingeo, G.; Del Campo, S.S.F.; Samouda, H.; La Frano, M.R.; Bohn, T. Strengthening the Immune System and Reducing Inflammation and Oxidative Stress through Diet and Nutrition: Considerations during the COVID-19 Crisis. *Nutrients* **2020**, *12*, 1562. [CrossRef]
60. Gonda, K.; Kanazawa, H.; Maeda, G.; Matayoshi, C.; Hirose, N.; Katsumoto, Y.; Kono, K.; Takenoshita, S. Ingestion of Okinawa Island Vegetables Increases IgA Levels and Prevents the Spread of Influenza RNA Viruses. *Nutrients* **2021**, *13*, 1773. [CrossRef] [PubMed]

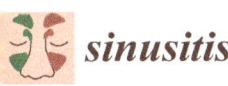

Review

Immunological and microRNA Features of Allergic Rhinitis in the Context of United Airway Disease

Kremena Naydenova [1], Vasil Dimitrov [1] and Tsvetelina Velikova [2,*]

1. Clinical Center of Allergology, University Hospital Alexandrovska, Department of Internal Medicine, Medical University of Sofia, Georgi Sofyiski 1 Str., 1431 Sofia, Bulgaria; kremenann@gmail.com (K.N.); vddim2012@gmail.com (V.D.)
2. Clinical Immunology, University Hospital Lozenetz, Sofia University St. Kliment Ohridski, 1407 Sofia, Bulgaria
* Correspondence: tsvelikova@medfac.mu-sofia.bg

Abstract: Inflammation of the upper respiratory tract in patients with allergic rhinitis (AR) may contribute to lower respiratory airways' inflammation. T-helper 17 (Th17) cells and related cytokines are also involved in the immunological mechanism of AR along with the classical Th2 cells. It is hypothesized that upon Th2 pressure, the inflammatory response in the lungs may lead to Th17-induced neutrophilic inflammation. However, the findings for interleukin-17 (IL-17) are bidirectional. Furthermore, the role of Th17 cells and their counterpart—T regulatory cells—remains unclear in AR patients. It was also shown that a regulator of inflammation might be the individual circulating specific non-coding microRNAs (miRNAs), which were distinctively expressed in AR and bronchial asthma (BA) patients. However, although several circulating miRNAs have been related to upper and lower respiratory tract diseases, their function and clinical value are far from being clarified. Still, they can serve as noninvasive biomarkers for diagnosing, characterizing, and providing therapeutic targets for anti-inflammatory treatment along with the confirmed contributors to the pathogenesis—Th17 cells and related cytokines. The narrow pathogenetic relationship between the nose and the bronchi, e.g., upper and lower respiratory tracts, confirms the concept of unified airway diseases. Thus, there is no doubt that AR and BA should be diagnosed, managed, and treated in an integrated manner.

Keywords: allergic rhinitis; bronchial asthma; allergy; Th17 cells; IL-17; IL-33; microRNA; miR; airway mucosal inflammation; united airway disease

Citation: Naydenova, K.; Dimitrov, V.; Velikova, T. Immunological and microRNA Features of Allergic Rhinitis in the Context of United Airway Disease. *Sinusitis* **2021**, *5*, 45–52. https://doi.org/10.3390/sinusitis5010005

Received: 10 December 2020
Accepted: 15 February 2021
Published: 19 February 2021

Publisher's Note: MDPI stays neutral with regard to jurisdictional claims in published maps and institutional affiliations.

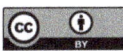

Copyright: © 2021 by the authors. Licensee MDPI, Basel, Switzerland. This article is an open access article distributed under the terms and conditions of the Creative Commons Attribution (CC BY) license (https://creativecommons.org/licenses/by/4.0/).

1. Introduction

The evidence gathered suggests a link between the upper and lower airways, grouped as "united airway, one disease" [1–5]. The topic is critical, and the interest and involvement of the specialists are continuously increasing.

Several mechanisms explain this connection. It is well known that the nose and sinuses have a significant protective function for the respiratory tract by warming, humidifying, and purifying the inhaled air. Any condition or disease affecting the upper respiratory tract's mucosal layer impedes this protection. This leads to exposing the lower respiratory tract to the harmful effects of polluted air, irritants, and allergens [6]. Therefore, patients suffering from allergic rhinitis (AR), sinusitis, and/or nasal polyposis may exhibit airway inflammation along with bronchial hyper-reactivity. Nasal and sinus involvement is closely related to bronchial asthma at both pathophysiological and clinical levels [1,2].

This review aims to reveal the recent advances in the "united airway disease pathway," focusing on allergic rhinitis, rhinosinusitis, and other airway conditions, such as bronchial hyper-reactivity and allergic asthma. Along with the common pathophysiology, the upper and lower airway diseases share common diagnostic and treatment approaches. This is especially valid when multiple conditions present simultaneously.

2. Allergic Rhinitis in the Continuum of Airway Inflammation

One of the most common allergic diseases is AR, affecting up to 40% of the population [7]. The prevalence in the Bulgarian population is 18.2%, as shown in a 2000 study [8]. The disease is IgE-mediated and non-infectious, affecting the nasal mucosa. The condition may involve the conjunctiva in 70–75% of cases after contact with environmental allergens [9]. Although AR is not a life-threatening disease, it significantly impairs patients' quality of life and the efficiency of daily activities [10].

Approximately 40% of patients have comorbidities such as bronchial asthma (BA), while most patients with BA (85–90%) also have concomitant AR [11]. In patients with BA, the inflammation affecting the nose and sinuses shares common pathological features with that of the lungs [1,10].

It is worth mentioning that in nasal polyposis, the inflammation is predominantly eosinophilic with local production of IgE antibodies [12]. Furthermore, nasal polyps formed by the mucosa's growth in the paranasal sinuses and that prolapse into the nasal cavity contribute to the nasal obstruction. In clinical practice, the simultaneous presence of BA, polyposis, and aspirin sensitivity is referred to as Samter's triad, or aspirin-exacerbated respiratory disease [13]. This is another proof of the united airway pathway concept.

3. Upper Airway Cough Syndrome

The relationship between the upper and lower respiratory tracts can be represented with the common symptom of coughing. The latter remains a diagnostic and treatment challenge in clinical practice. Upper respiratory tract infections play a significant role as a risk factor in the development of asthma. Moreover, they are the most common identified cause of chronic cough in adults [14]. Inflammation is common among chronic diseases characterized by coughing. Usually, the inflammatory process is spread from the upper to the lower respiratory tract [15].

In line with this, chronic inflammation that affects the upper and lower respiratory tracts is referred to as sinobronchial syndrome [16]. This syndrome includes chronic rhinosinusitis together with nonspecific inflammation of the lower airways (e.g., chronic bronchitis, bronchiectasis, and diffuse panbronchiolitis). It has been hypothesized that sinusitis occurs first, then the inflammation progresses to bronchial disease. Clinically, markers of bronchial irritation usually correlate with sinusitis severity. This hypothesis assumes that postnasal drip entering the trachea plays an essential role in developing the disease [17,18]. The anatomical relation between the upper and lower airways suggests the possible involvement of nasal discharge to provoke bronchial hyper-reactivity in patients with AR or rhinosinusitis [19]. As postnasal drip is not a diagnosis but a symptom, a broad differential diagnosis should be made, including AR, vasomotor rhinitis, viral or bacterial infections, and nasal polyps [20].

Upper airway cough syndrome (UACS) is the cause of chronic cough in 18.6–67% of cases in China [21]. Cough in patients with UACS is usually secondary due to upper airway diseases (i.e., affecting the nose and sinuses). Pekova et al. reported increased cough sensitivity in patients with AR without cough relative to healthy controls' sensitivity to cough. The difference between the two groups was predominantly pronounced during the pollen season. Nevertheless, the cough hypersensitivity syndrome observed in allergic patients may be one of the mechanisms leading to cough in patients with UACS [22].

Cough hypersensitivity to capsaicin in patients with allergic asthma increases during the birch pollen season. Increased sensitivity was observed with prolonged pollen exposure in the same patients. This observation suggests that allergic inflammation of the lower and/or the upper respiratory tract stimulates neurogenic mechanisms of significant clinical importance [23]. Explanations include that patients with AR may have an increased number of neurons that release large amounts of neuroinflammatory mediators in the nasal mucosa. Inflammatory mediators not only activate sensory neurons but also sensitize them, lowering their activation threshold.

Kaiser et al. [24] studied neuropeptides' levels in nasal secretions in patients with and without chronic cough. They found that patients with cough and postnasal drip had significantly higher levels of neuropeptides, such as calcitonin gene-related peptide (CGRP) and substance P (SP), compared to patients without complaints. This study supports and confirms the role of neuropeptides in increased nasopharyngeal discharge and cough hypersensitivity in the context of the united airway disease.

4. Immune Cells Involved in United Airway Inflammation

It was previously established that to maintain immune homeostasis, it is vital to obtain a balance between the regulatory and effectors immune cells, such as T-helper type 1 (Th1) and type 2 (Th2) cells. As the Th1/Th2 balance dysregulates, the released cytokines contribute to the development of chronic inflammation of the mucosa, resulting in autoimmune or allergic diseases [25].

It is assumed that AR is related to the first type of allergic sensitization in Coombs' classification, where the involvement of IgE antibodies is crucial [26]. Early and late phases of an allergic response are observed.

Briefly, the immunological mechanism can be represented as follows: upon contact with the mucosa, the allergen is taken up by the antigen-presenting cells, which process it and present it to Th2 cells. Activated Th2 lymphocytes release IL-4, IL-6, IL-13, etc., which interact with B lymphocytes. This interaction leads to the activation of B cells and the synthesis of specific IgE antibodies. IgE antibodies bind to their high-affinity receptors on mast cells' surfaces and, upon contact with the specific allergen, lead to cell degranulation. As a result, several mediators are released, such as histamine, leukotrienes, and prostaglandins. This description represents the early phase of an allergic response observed within the first few minutes after the allergen contact that lasts 2–3 h.

In the late phase, which occurs 4–6 h after antigenic stimulation, cellular infiltration of the mucosa consists mainly of T lymphocytes, eosinophils, and basophils. In the described Th2 response, IgE antibody production requires two main signals to switch B cells to an IgE antibody-producing plasma cell. The first signal is provided by the cytokines IL-4 or IL-13, which interact with B cell receptors. They transmit the signal by activating the tyrosine kinases of the Janus family— Janus kinase 1 (JAK1) and JAK3—which leads to phosphorylation of the STAT6 transcription regulator. The second signal for IgE switching is additional stimulation by contact between the CD40 ligand on the T cell surface and CD40 on the B cell surface [27]. It is worth mentioning that the allergen stimulation of the immune system leads to priming of the entire mucosa of the airways.

Nasal polyps are also rich in inflammatory immune cells, such as eosinophils, Th lymphocytes, plasma cells, and mast cells. Histologically, nasal polyps are characterized by an edematous stroma, eosinophilia, a thickened basement membrane, and a damaged ciliary epithelium. It is not surprising that chronic inflammation in the nasal polyps, allergic or not, resembles the bronchial mucosa inflammation observed in asthma. This once again confirms the united disease pathways of the airways. Nevertheless, in 30–70% of patients with nasal polyposis, accompanying BA is diagnosed [28].

Interestingly, it was shown that AR without polyposis or eosinophilic inflammation may not possess the common airway pathways with asthma, unlike the case where all present together [29]. Taken together, data on the united airway pathway suggest that AR should be seen as predictive risk factor for asthma [30].

5. Th17 Cells Role in the Common Inflammation of the Airways

In recent decades, discovering Th17 cells and regulatory T (Treg) cells has dramatically complicated the established Th1/Th2 paradigm. Involvement of the two counterparts—Th17 cells and Tregs—complicates the understanding of AR's pathogenesis [31]. The role of Th17 cells in neutrophil infiltration and chronic inflammation in AR and asthma is well established. Moreover, it was confirmed that the balance between Th17/Treg cells matters clinically in allergic and autoimmune diseases.

Speaking of the united airway pathway, the participation of Th17 in the pathogenesis and progression of AR and other diseases is also proven. Moreover, a correlation of IL-17 levels in the inflamed airway mucosa with the severity of the allergic disease was found [32].

Many studies have proven the involvement of Th17 cells and IL-17 in the immunological mechanism of AR. A recent study by Huang et al. [33] examined Th17/Treg cells immunity in AR patients. The results showed that Th17 cells were significantly increased in the peripheral blood of patients with AR, whereas the Treg cell number was decreased. The results suggested that the Th17/Treg imbalance plays a crucial role in AR's pathogenesis and severity.

Moreover, Milovanovic et al. demonstrated that IL-17 could induce B cell switching to IgE antibody production, endorsing, once again, the involvement of Th17 in allergic diseases [34]. However, Th17 cells produce a large number of mediators, but IL-17A can directly induce IgE production.

A schematic picture of the immune mediators and cells involved in the airway mucosa inflammation is presented in Figure 1.

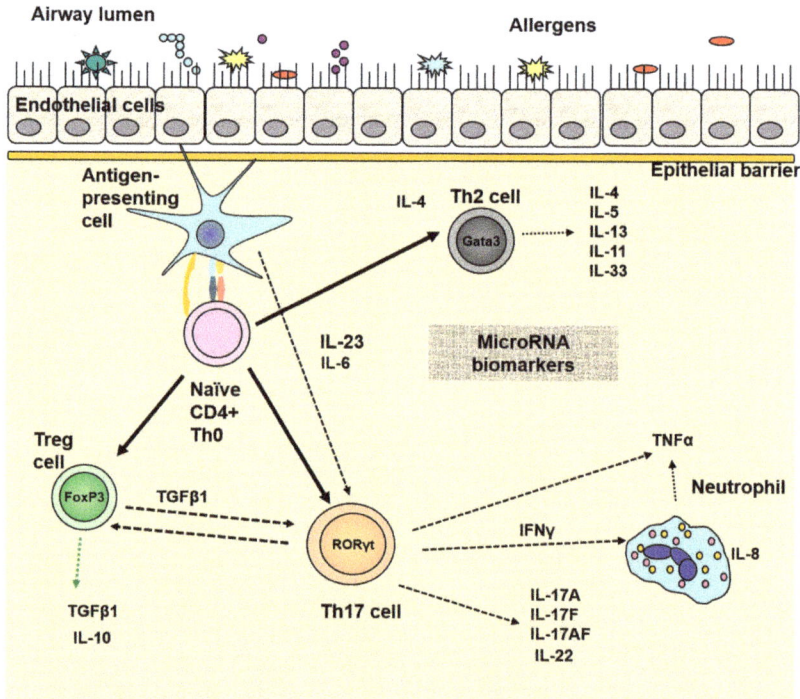

Figure 1. Immunological interactions in the inflamed mucosa in the concept of united airway disease. Naïve T cells differentiate either into Th2, Tregs, or Th17 cells. By secreting a distinct array of cytokines, Th17, Th2, and Treg cells connect innate and adaptive immune responses in the airway mucosa, especially during mucosal inflammation. Balance of Th17/Tegs is needed to maintain the immune homeostasis in the mucosa and to resolve the inflammation. Note: allergens are presented as different shaped objects in the airway lumen.

Another cytokine with a role in the common airway inflammation and allergic diseases is IL-33. It is a member of the IL-1 cytokine family released in response to epithelial cell damage. IL-33 exerts many actions by interacting with the suppressor of tumorigenicity 2 (ST2) receptor. Furthermore, it can induce Th2 cytokine-mediated allergic inflammation [35].

The IL-33/ST2-induced Th2 response has been found to interact with the Th17 immune response in AR pathology [36,37]. IL-33 also induces the production of proinflammatory cytokines and participates in the pathogenesis of diseases other than AR, such as atopic dermatitis, BA, and pollinosis.

The crucial role of IL-33 in the united airway inflammation is based on bridging the innate and acquired immune responses in allergic diseases [38]. Clinically, this connection was evaluated by the reported correlation of IL-33 levels and the AR severity [39].

Other cytokines, such as those with anti-inflammatory properties—IL-10, TGF-β, and IL-35—and related to Th17 and Th22 cells—IL-22 and IL-27—might shape the allergic responses as well. Still, there are few reports on their role [40]. The cytokines related to Th17 and Treg activation while suppressing Th1 cells—IL-17, IL-22, and TGF-β—were found enhanced in AR patients. On the contrary, IL-35, which was shown to inhibit both Th2- and Th17-mediated allergic airway inflammation, was detected low in patients with AR, showing the possible role in the pathogenesis of allergic diseases [40].

6. Diagnostic and Therapeutic Approaches in the Light of the United Airway Pathway

By enhancing the understanding of the inflammation of the upper respiratory tract and the pathogenesis of AR and other allergic diseases, new diagnostic and therapeutic approaches can be established. They can facilitate the management and follow-up of the patients and improve their quality of life.

6.1. microRNAs as a Promising Tool in United Airway Disease Diagnosis

Promising and advanced tools for diagnosing and managing patients with AR and BA are the small non-coding RNAs, known as microRNAs (miRNA or miR). As specific gene expression regulators, miRNAs regulate many biological processes, including cell differentiation, proliferation, and survival [41]. Furthermore, they can serve as noninvasive biomarkers for diagnosis, molecular classification, severity, and relapse prediction [38]. miRNAs tend to participate in the pathogenesis of both AR and BA. It was shown that individual circulating miRNAs were distinctively expressed in AR and BA patients [42].

Moreover, few studies examined their role in clinical settings. Suojalehto et al. found increased levels of miR-143, miR-187, miR-498, miR-874, and miR-886-3p and decreased levels of let-7e, miR-18a, miR-126, miR-155, and miR-224 in BA compared to controls [42]. However, these results were independent of concomitant AR. Thus, no distinction was made between BA and AR based on these expressions.

In the second study, Suojalehto et al. [43] found upregulated expression of miR-155, miR-205, and miR-498 but downregulated expression of let-7e in the nasal mucosa of AR patients and current symptoms in comparison with AR without asthma. However, the cytokine levels (IL-4, IL-5, and IL-13) and miRNA expression profile were comparable in AR with or without AB, suggesting that concomitant asthma might have a minor impact.

In addition, an alternative to the nonsteroidal anti-inflammatory treatment, adjusting and regulating the miRNA network, may be a promising therapy approach.

6.2. Biological Therapy in the Focus of United Airway Disease

The success of all available treatment strategies for united airway disease relies on the combined targeting of all clinically presented diseases. The similar pathological pathways and common mucosal inflammation, along with the parallel incidence of AR and BA, lead to the approach for similar treatment, including biological therapy, as we showed previously [44–47].

The strategy of using biological agents has been investigated in patients with AR, BA, and other allergic diseases. Biological therapy was considered a beneficial treatment option in patients with severe uncontrolled phenotypes of diseases. Omalizumab, which represents a humanized anti-IgE monoclonal antibody, has been studied extensively for AR and BA. It confirmed its effectiveness in preventing IgE to attach to its high-affinity receptors. Moreover, omalizumab's clinical outcomes have been linked to reducing nasal and asthma symptoms, decreasing the number of exacerbations by affecting both the upper and lower airways [47]. All of these led to an overall improvement in the quality of life of the patients.

Another monoclonal antibody used for both AR and BA—mepolizumab—acts by blocking the binding of IL-5 to eosinophils. Mepolizumab has also shown efficacy in improving the severity of eosinophilic airway diseases, especially in BA and nasal polyps [48,49].

Nevertheless, we must always have in mind that monoclonal therapy is not without systemic effects. In line with this, in patients with united airway disease due to the effects of therapy on AR improvement, it is hardly possible to design a study to distinguish the improvement in BA alone. In line with this, management of AR and BA must be carried out together to obtain better control of both diseases [50].

7. Conclusions

The concept of unified airway diseases has been the subject of attention in recent years. The pathogenetic relationship of the nose and the bronchi and alveoli, along with the observed common inflammation, provides a niche to create new diagnostic and therapeutic options.

With Th17 cells and other immune cells and mediators, gene alteration and regulation by miRNA complicate the picture of the united airway inflammation. More research here is needed to better understand the associations between the upper and lower airways. However, there is no doubt that AR and BA should be diagnosed, managed, and treated in an integrated manner.

Author Contributions: Conceptualization, K.N. and T.V.; writing—original draft preparation, K.N.; writing—review and editing, T.V.; visualization, T.V.; supervision, V.D. All authors have read and agreed to the published version of the manuscript.

Funding: This research received no external funding.

Institutional Review Board Statement: Not applicable.

Informed Consent Statement: Not applicable.

Data Availability Statement: Not applicable.

Conflicts of Interest: The authors declare no conflict of interest.

References

1. Caimmi, D.; Marseglia, A.; Pieri, G.; Benzo, S.; Bosa, L.; Caimmi, S. Nose and lungs: One way, one disease. *Ital. J. Pediatr.* **2012**, *38*, 60. [CrossRef] [PubMed]
2. Licari, A.; Castagnoli, R.; Denicolò, C.F.; Rossini, L.; Marseglia, A.; Marseglia, G.L. The Nose and the Lung: United Airway Disease? *Front. Pediatr.* **2017**, *5*, 44. [CrossRef]
3. Haccuria, A.; van Muylem, A.; Malinovschi, A.; Doan, V.; Michils, A. Small airways dysfunction: The link between allergic rhinitis and allergic asthma. *Eur. Respir. J.* **2018**, *51*, 1701749. [CrossRef]
4. Compalati, E.; Ridolo, E.; Passalacqua, G.; Braido, F.; Villa, E.; Canonica, G.W. The link between allergic rhinitis and asthma: The united airways disease. *Expert Rev. Clin. Immunol.* **2010**, *6*, 413–423. [CrossRef]
5. Vujnovic, S.D.; Domuz, A. Epidemiological Aspects of Rhinitis and Asthma: Comorbidity or United Airway Disease. In *Asthma Diagnosis and Management—Approach Based on Phenotype and Endotype*; IntechOpen: London, UK, 2018.
6. Bousquet, J.; Boushey, H.A.; Busse, W.W.; Canonica, G.W.; Durham, S.R.; Irvin, C.G.; Karpel, J.P.; van Cauwenberge, P.; Chen, R.; Iezzoni, D.G.; et al. Characteristics of patients with seasonal allergic rhinitis and concomitant asthma. *Clin. Exp. Allergy* **2004**, *34*, 897–903. [CrossRef]
7. Small, P.; Keith, P.K.; Kim, H. Allergic rhinitis. *Allergy Asthma Clin. Immunol.* **2018**, *14*, 1–11. [CrossRef] [PubMed]
8. Mileva, Z.; Popov, T.; Staneva, M.; Dimitrov, V.; Mateev, V.; Slavov, S. Frequency and characteristics of allergic diseases in Bulgaria. *Allergy Asthma* **2000**, *1*, 3–32.
9. Pawankar, R.; Bunnag, C.; Khaltaev, N.; Bousquet, J. Allergic Rhinitis and Its Impact on Asthma in Asia Pacific and the ARIA Update 2008. *World Allergy Organ. J.* **2012**, *5*, S212–S217. [CrossRef]
10. Dykewicz, M.S. 7. Rhinitis and sinusitis. *J. Allergy Clin. Immunol.* **2003**, *111*, S520–S529. [CrossRef] [PubMed]

11. Bousquet, P.; Schünemann, H.; Samolinski, B.; Demoly, P.; Baena-Cagnani, C.; Bachert, C.; Bonini, S.; Boulet, L.; Brozek, J.; Canonica, G.; et al. Allergic Rhinitis and its Impact on Asthma (ARIA): Achievements in 10 years and future needs. *J. Allergy Clin. Immunol.* **2012**, *130*, 1049–1062. [CrossRef] [PubMed]
12. Bugten, V.; Nordgård, S.; Romundstad, P.; Steinsvåg, S. Chronic rhinosinusitis and nasal polyposis; indicia of heterogeneity. *Rhinol. J.* **2008**, *46*, 40–44.
13. Ediger, D.; Sin, B.A.; Heper, A.; Anadolu, Y.; Mitoasitoarlitoagil, Z. Airway inflammation in nasal polyposis: Immunopathological aspects of relation to asthma. *Clin. Exp. Allergy* **2005**, *35*, 319–326. [CrossRef]
14. Bousquet, J.; van Cauwenberge, P.; Khaltaev, N. Allergic Rhinitis and Its Impact on Asthma. *J. Allergy Clin. Immunol.* **2001**, *108*, S147–S334. [CrossRef]
15. Millqvist, E.; Bende, M. Role of the upper airways in patients with chronic cough. *Curr. Opin. Allergy Clin. Immunol.* **2006**, *6*, 7–11. [CrossRef] [PubMed]
16. Kogahara, T.; Kanai, K.-I.; Asano, K.; Suzaki, H. Evidence for passing down of postnasal drip into respiratory organs. *Vivo* **2009**, *23*, 297–302.
17. Pratter, M.R. Chronic Upper Airway Cough Syndrome Secondary to Rhinosinus Diseases (Previously Referred to as Postnasal Drip Syndrome). *Chest* **2006**, *129*, 63S–71S. [CrossRef]
18. Forer, M.; Ananda, S. The management of postnasal drip. *Aust. Fam. Physician* **1999**, *28*, 223–228. [PubMed]
19. Meltzer, E.O.; Szwarcberg, J.; Pill, M.W. Allergic Rhinitis, Asthma, and Rhinosinusitis: Diseases of the Integrated Airway. *J. Manag. Care Pharm.* **2004**, *10*, 310–317. [CrossRef]
20. Morice, A.H. The diagnosis and management of chronic cough. *Eur. Respir. J.* **2004**, *24*, 481–492. [CrossRef] [PubMed]
21. Lai, K.; Chen, R.; Lin, J.; Huang, K.; Shen, H.; Kong, L.; Zhou, X.; Luo, Z.; Yang, L.; Wen, F.; et al. A Prospective, Multicenter Survey on Causes of Chronic Cough in China. *Chest* **2013**, *143*, 613–620. [CrossRef]
22. Pecova, R.; Zucha, J.; Pec, M.; Neuschlova, M.; Hanzel, P.; Tatar, M. Cough reflex sensitivity testing in in seasonal allergic rhinitis patients and healthy volunteers. *J. Physiol. Pharmacol.* **2008**, *59*, 557–564. [PubMed]
23. Weinfeld, D.; Ternesten-Hasséus, E.; Löwhagen, O.; Millqvist, E. Capsaicin cough sensitivity in allergic asthmatic patients increases during the birch pollen season. *Ann. Allergy Asthma Immunol.* **2002**, *89*, 419–424. [CrossRef]
24. Lim, K.G.; Rank, M.A.; Kita, H.; Patel, A.; Moore, E. Neuropeptide levels in nasal secretions from patients with and without chronic cough. *Ann. Allergy Asthma Immunol.* **2011**, *107*, 360–363. [CrossRef] [PubMed]
25. Romagnani, S. T-cell subsets (Th1 versus Th2). *Ann. Allergy Asthma Immunol.* **2000**, *85*, 9–21. [CrossRef]
26. Rajan, T. The Gell—Coombs classification of hypersensitivity reactions: A re-interpretation. *Trends Immunol.* **2003**, *24*, 376–379. [CrossRef]
27. Janeway, C.A., Jr.; Travers, P.; Walport, M.; Shlomchik, M.J. *Immunobiology: The Immune System in Health and Disease*, 5th ed.; Garland Science: New York, NY, USA, 2001.
28. Larsen, K. The Clinical Relationship of Nasal Polyps to Asthma. *Allergy Asthma Proc.* **1996**, *17*, 243–249. [CrossRef]
29. Muluk, N.B. The united airway disease. *Rom. J. Rhinol.* **2019**, *9*, 1–26. [CrossRef]
30. Ketenci, A.; Kalyoncu, A.F.; del Giacco, S. Upper and Lower Airways Interaction: Is the United Airway Disease Concept a Reflection of Reality? How Important Is It? In *Challenges in Rhinology*; Cingi, C., Muluk, N.B., Scadding, G.K., Mladina, R., Eds.; Springer International Publishing: Cham, Switzerland, 2020; pp. 405–414.
31. Gu, Z.W.; Wang, Y.X.; Cao, Z.W. Neutralization of interleukin-17 suppresses allergic rhinitis symptoms by downregulating Th2 and Th17 responses and upregulating the Treg response. *Oncotarget* **2017**, *8*, 22361–22369. [CrossRef]
32. Ciprandi, G.; de Amici, M.; Murdaca, G.; Fenoglio, D.; Ricciardolo, F.L.M.; Marseglia, G.L.; Tosca, M. Serum interleukin-17 levels are related to clinical severity in allergic rhinitis. *Allergy* **2009**, *64*, 1375–1378. [CrossRef] [PubMed]
33. Huang, X.; Chen, Y.; Zhang, F.; Yang, Q.; Zhang, G. Peripheral Th17/Treg cell-mediated immunity imbalance in allergic rhinitis patients. *Braz. J. Otorhinolaryngol.* **2014**, *80*, 152–155. [CrossRef] [PubMed]
34. Ferretti, E.; di Carlo, E.; Ognio, E.; Guarnotta, C.; Bertoni, F.; Corcione, A.; Prigione, I.; Fraternali-Orcioni, G.; Ribatti, D.; Ravetti, J.L.; et al. Interleukin-17A promotes the growth of human germinal center derived non-Hodgkin B cell lymphoma. *OncoImmunology* **2015**, *4*, e1030560. [CrossRef]
35. Haenuki, Y.; Matsushita, K.; Futatsugi-Yumikura, S.; Ishii, K.J.; Kawagoe, T.; Imoto, Y.; Fujieda, S.; Yasuda, M.; Hisa, Y.; Akira, S.; et al. A critical role of IL-33 in experimental allergic rhinitis. *J. Allergy Clin. Immunol.* **2012**, *130*, 184–194.e11. [CrossRef] [PubMed]
36. Vocca, L.; di Sano, C.; Uasuf, C.G.; Sala, A.; Riccobono, L.; Gangemi, S.; Albano, G.D.; Bonanno, A.; Gagliardo, R.; Profita, M. IL-33/ST2 axis controls Th2/IL-31 and Th17 immune response in allergic airway diseases. *Immunobiology* **2015**, *220*, 954–963. [CrossRef]
37. Ding, W.; Zou, G.-L.; Zhang, W.; Lai, X.-N.; Chen, H.-W.; Xiong, L.-X. Interleukin-33: Its Emerging Role in Allergic Diseases. *Molecules* **2018**, *23*, 1665. [CrossRef]
38. Lloyd, C.M. IL-33 family members and asthma—Bridging innate and adaptive immune responses. *Curr. Opin. Immunol.* **2010**, *22*, 800–806. [CrossRef]
39. Glück, J.; Rymarczyk, B.; Rogala, B. Serum IL-33 but not ST2 level is elevated in intermittent allergic rhinitis and is a marker of the disease severity. *Inflamm. Res.* **2012**, *61*, 547–550. [CrossRef]

40. Degirmenci, P.B.; Aksun, S.; Altin, Z.; Bilgir, F.; Arslan, I.B.; Çolak, H.; Ural, B.; Kahraman, D.S.; Diniz, G.; Ozdemir, B.; et al. Allergic Rhinitis and Its Relationship with IL-10, IL-17, TGF-β, IFN-γ, IL 22, and IL-35. *Dis. Markers* **2018**, *2018*, 1–6. [CrossRef] [PubMed]
41. Liu, Z.; Zhang, X.-H.; Callejas-Díaz, B.; Mullol, J. MicroRNA in United Airway Diseases. *Int. J. Mol. Sci.* **2016**, *17*, 716. [CrossRef] [PubMed]
42. Panganiban, R.P.; Wang, Y.; Howrylak, J.; Chinchilli, V.M.; Craig, T.J.; August, A.; Ishmael, F.T. Circulating microRNAs as biomarkers in patients with allergic rhinitis and asthma. *J. Allergy Clin. Immunol.* **2016**, *137*, 1423–1432. [CrossRef]
43. Suojalehto, H.; Lindström, I.; Majuri, M.-L.; Mitts, C.; Karjalainen, J.; Wolff, H.; Alenius, H. Altered MicroRNA Expression of Nasal Mucosa in Long-Term Asthma and Allergic Rhinitis. *Int. Arch. Allergy Immunol.* **2014**, *163*, 168–178. [CrossRef]
44. Naydenova, K.; Velikova, T.; Dimitrov, V. Interactions of allergic rhinitis and bronchial asthma at mucosal immunology level. *AIMS Allergy Immunol.* **2019**, *3*, 1–12. [CrossRef]
45. Naydenova, K.; Velikova, T.V.; Dimitrov, V. Chapter 5. Allergic Rhinitis, IL-17 and the Concept of a Common Respiratory Pathway. In *Th17 Cells in Health and Disease*; Nova Publishing: New York, NY, USA, 2020.
46. Naydenova, K.; Velikova, T.V.; Dimitrov, V. Mucosal Inflammation in Allergic Rhinitis and Bronchial Asthma—Two Sides of a Coin. *Clin. Res. Immunol.* **2018**, *1*, 1–2.
47. Gevaert, P.; Calus, L.; van Zele, T.; Blomme, K.; de Ruyck, N.; Bauters, W.; Hellings, P.; Brusselle, G.; de Bacquer, D.; van Cauwenberge, P.; et al. Omalizumab is effective in allergic and nonallergic patients with nasal polyps and asthma. *J. Allergy Clin. Immunol.* **2013**, *131*, 110–116.e1. [CrossRef] [PubMed]
48. Pavord, I.D.; Korn, S.; Howarth, P.; Bleecker, E.R.; Buhl, R.; Keene, O.N.; Ortega, H.; Chanez, P. Mepolizumab for severe eosinophilic asthma (DREAM): A multicentre, double-blind, placebo-controlled trial. *Lancet* **2012**, *380*, 651–659. [CrossRef]
49. Gevaert, P.; van Bruaene, N.; Cattaert, T.; van Steen, K.; van Zele, T.; Acke, F.; de Ruyck, N.; Blomme, K.; Sousa, A.R.; Marshall, R.P.; et al. Mepolizumab, a humanized anti–IL-5 mAb, as a treatment option for severe nasal polyposis. *J. Allergy Clin. Immunol.* **2011**, *128*, 989–995.e8. [CrossRef]
50. Giavina-Bianchi, P.; Aun, M.V.; Takejima, P.; Kalil, J.; Agondi, R.C. United airway disease: Current perspectives. *J. Asthma Allergy* **2016**, *9*, 93–100. [CrossRef] [PubMed]

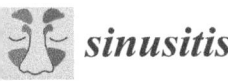

Article

Anti-Asthmatic Effects of Saffron Extract and Salbutamol in an Ovalbumin-Induced Airway Model of Allergic Asthma

Pranav Nair and Kedar Prabhavalkar *

Department of Pharmacology, SVKM's Dr. Bhanuben Nanavati College of Pharmacy, Vile Parle (W), Mumbai 400056, India; pranavam95@gmail.com
* Correspondence: kspharmac@gmail.com

Abstract: Introduction: Asthma is a chronic inflammatory disorder of the airways often characterized by airway remodeling and influx of inflammatory cells into the airways. Saffron *(C. sativus)* has been reported to possess anti-inflammatory, anti-allergic and immunomodulatory properties. Salbutamol is known to relax airway smooth muscles. Objective: To investigate the combined anti-asthmatic effect of *C. sativus* extract (CSE) and salbutamol in an ovalbumin (OVA)-induced asthma in rats. Materials and methods: Airway hyperresponsiveness (AHR) was induced in male Sprague-Dawley rats by OVA challenge and treated with CSE (30 mg/kg and 60 mg/kg i.p.) and salbutamol (0.5 mg/kg p.o) for 28 days. After the induction period, various hematological, biochemical, molecular (ELISA) and histological analyses were performed. Results: OVA-induced alterations observed in hematological parameters (total and differential cell counts observed in Bronchoalveolar Lavage Fluid (BALF) were significantly attenuated ($p < 0.01$) by CSE (30 mg/kg and 60 mg/kg) and salbutamol (0.5 mg/kg). The treatment combination also significantly decreased ($p < 0.01$) the levels of total protein and albumin in serum, BALF and lung tissues. Treatment with CSE and salbutamol significantly attenuated ($p < 0.01$) increase in OVA induced Th2 cytokine levels (TNF-α, IL-1β, IL-4, IL-13). Histopathological analysis of lung tissue showed that combined effect of CSE and salbutamol treatment ameliorated OVA-induced inflammatory influx and ultrastructural aberrations. Conclusion: The results obtained from this study show that the combined effect of CSE and salbutamol exhibited anti-asthmatic properties via its anti-inflammatory effect and by alleviating Th2 mediated immune response. Thus, this treatment combination could be considered as a new therapeutic strategy for management of asthma.

Keywords: asthma; ovalbumin; saffron; salbutamol; IL's; TNF-α

Citation: Nair, P.; Prabhavalkar, K. Anti-Asthmatic Effects of Saffron Extract and Salbutamol in an Ovalbumin-Induced Airway Model of Allergic Asthma. *Sinusitis* 2021, 5, 17–31. https://doi.org/10.3390/sinusitis5010003

Received: 26 October 2020
Accepted: 14 January 2021
Published: 24 January 2021

Publisher's Note: MDPI stays neutral with regard to jurisdictional claims in published maps and institutional affiliations.

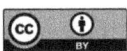

Copyright: © 2021 by the authors. Licensee MDPI, Basel, Switzerland. This article is an open access article distributed under the terms and conditions of the Creative Commons Attribution (CC BY) license (https://creativecommons.org/licenses/by/4.0/).

1. Introduction

Amongst chronic respiratory diseases, chronic obstructive pulmonary disease (COPD) and asthma are the leading cause of mortality worldwide [1]. Asthma is a complex heterogeneous chronic disease that affects people of diverse age groups. It is characterized by three main features: (1) Chronic inflammation of the airways (2) Variable airflow obstruction (3) Airway hyperresponsiveness (AHR). Other characteristic features include airway constriction, increased mucus production, reversible bronchospasm, multicellular inflammation and airway remodeling.

Inflammatory mediators such as eosinophils, neutrophils, mast cells, T lymphocytes, and dendritic cells play a major role in the development of asthma [2]. Acute lung inflammation followed by lung injury leads to pulmonary fibrosis, which in turn impairs gas exchange. Influx of eosinophils into the airways can cause epithelial damage, exudation of plasma wall, airway wall and basement membrane thickening [3,4].

Various treatment strategies have been devised for effective management and treatment of asthma. These include inhaled Bronchoprovocation challenges, corticosteroids, mast cell stabilizers, β2 adrenergic agonists, anti cholinergics, antihistamines, leukotriene modifiers etc. [5] Corticosteroids along with bronchodilators are the treatment of choice for severe asthmatics. Various studies involving dexamethasone has failed to show significant improvement in respiratory clinical score or hospital admission rate, whereas according to a meta-analysis, beta2-agonists failed to improve clinical symptoms when compared with a placebo [6,7]. In another study, no improvement was observed when dexamethasone, salbutamol, epinephrine was given alone in a similar set of population [8]. However, combination therapy involving dexamethasone and salbutamol has reported an improvement in hospital admission rate or respiratory clinical score when compared with placebo. Although the exact mechanism of action for this combination therapy is unknown, synergism between these two classes of drugs is well documented. Reports suggest that this combination of drugs showed a synergistic effect in children with bronchiolitis [6,8]. Patients experience different comorbidities due to prolong use of different corticosteroids. Hence it is imperative to find a substitute that can replace or to certain extent diminish the side effects associated with corticosteroids.

However, the current treatment regimen largely aims to decrease the symptoms and improve lung function by decreasing airway inflammation and restoring normal lung functions. Despite this, only a fraction of patients receives symptomatic relief. Side effects associated with these treatment strategies are a major concern. Thus, there is a need to develop medications that are not only efficacious but are also safe at the same time [5].

Saffron *(C. Sativus)* along with salbutamol could be considered as a potential drug to substitute corticosteroids because of its immunomodulatory, anti-inflammatory and airway smooth muscle relaxing effects. The present study aims to investigate the combined effect of saffron extract and Salbutamol in an ovalbumin-induced rat model of asthma.

2. Material and methods

2.1. Preparation of C. sativus Extract (CSE)

C. sativus extract (CSE) was prepared according to the method previously described [9]. An ultrasound-assisted extraction was performed in order to obtain the CSE. Saffron petals were crushed into powder and suspended in distilled water containing 0.3% Tween-80. This suspension was sonicated for 10 min in an ultrasound water bath (water temperature at 25 °C) and was passed through a 0.45 μm filter. The resulting solution (CSE) was then administered intraperitoneally (i.p.) in a volume of 0.5 mL per rat.

2.2. Animals

Healthy Sprague Dawley rats with a weight range of 180–200 g were procured from National Institute of Biosciences. They were housed in Perspex cages and maintained under standard laboratory conditions (12 h: 12 h dark—light cycle, a temperature of (24 ± 2 °C and 45–55% humidity. The animals were fed on standard food pellets and drinking water ad libitum. Before starting the experiment, animals were acclimatized for a period of one week. The entire experimental protocol was reviewed and approved by an Institutional Animal Ethics Committee registered under "Committee for the Purpose of Control and Supervision of Experiment on Laboratory Animals" (CPCSEA), Ministry of Environment and Forests, Government of India. Approval number—CPCSEA/IAEC/P-34/2018.

2.3. Chemicals

Ovalbumin (OVA, egg albumin grade II), and aluminum hydroxide were purchased from Sigma Chemical Co. (St Louis, MO), Salbutamol was purchased from TCI chemicals (Tokyo, Japan), Saffron was purchased from Yucca enterprises (Mumbai, India). Marketed preparation of Dexamethasone sodium phosphate was used (Martin & Brown Biosciences). All other purchases were made from S.D. fine chemicals (Mumbai, India).

2.4. Preparation of Crocus Sativus Extract (CSE):

Different Dosages of CSE Extract Was Freshly Prepared and Administered Intraperitoneally (i.p.) in a Volume of 0.5 mL per Rat. Salbutamol was Freshly Prepared Daily as 1% Aqueous Solution of Saline and Administered Orally at a Dose of 0.5 mg/kg [10]. Dexamethasone Sodium Phosphate (0.1 mg/kg) Was Administered as per Body Weight. Control Animals Received Isovolumetric Amounts (0.5 mL) of 0.3% Tween-80.

2.5. Induction of Asthma

Sensitization procedures and aerosol challenge were performed according to reported procedure with some minor changes [11]. Animals were actively sensitized by an intraperitoneal (i.p.) injection of 0.66 mL of a suspension of 1 mg OVA plus 300 mg of aluminum hydroxide in saline, this was considered as Day 0 of sensitization. Seven days after sensitization, the animals were boosted subcutaneously (s.c.) with an identical injection of aluminum-precipitated OVA in all the mentioned groups except normal control. The aluminum precipitate acts as an adjuvant to promote IgE production. The standard drugs and treatment drugs were administered daily for all 28 days in the standard and treatment groups, respectively. On day 28, intranasal (i.n.) OVA-aerosol challenge was accomplished by placing the rats individually in a polyurethane chamber connected to a nebulizer. This generated an aerosol mist pumped into the exposure chamber with an output volume of 10 mL. Except the Normal Control group, all other groups were exposed to 1% OVA-aerosol challenge for 15 min. Animals in normal control group were given saline aerosol for 15 min. On Day 29, 24 h after final OVA challenge (saline challenge for normal control group), the animals were anesthetized using urethane (1.25 g/kg) for collection of blood and Bronchoalveolar Lavage (BAL) fluid for biochemical evaluation. After that the animals were sacrificed, their lungs were isolated for further analyses. (Figure 1)

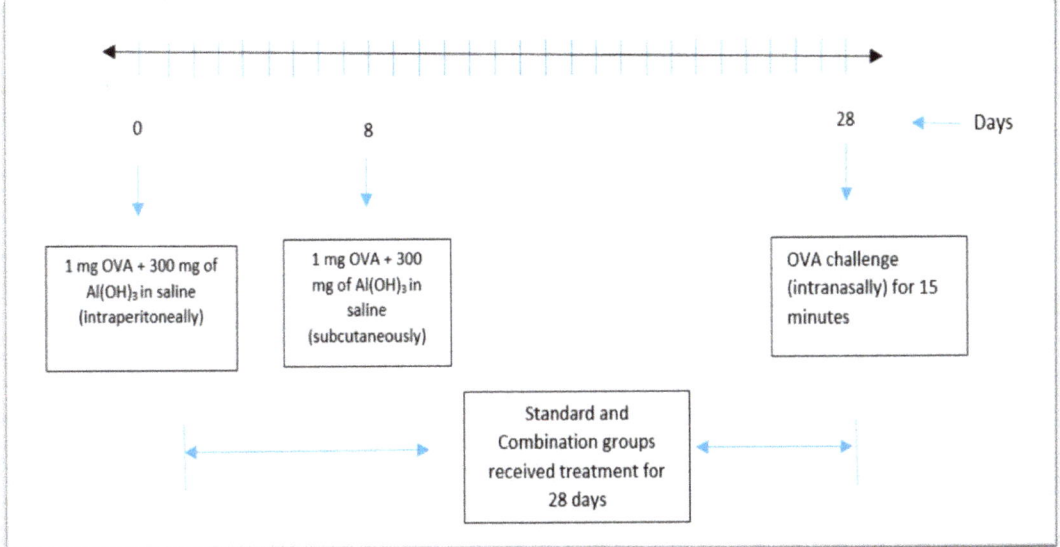

Figure 1. Timeline of the study.

Groups:

A. Normal Control—0.9% w/v saline
B. Negative control—1mg OVA + 300 mg Aluminium hydroxide
C. Standard—Dexamethasone (0.1 mg/kg) i.p + Salbutamol (0.5 mg/kg) oral
D. Combination 1—Saffron (30 mg/kg) i.p + Salbutamol (0.5 mg/kg) oral
E. Combination 2—Saffron (60 mg/kg) i.p + Salbutamol (0.5 mg/kg) oral

2.6. Determination of Cell Count in Blood

Blood (3 mL) was collected in a heparinized tube from each animal under anesthesia (urethane (1.25 mg/kg)) and used for leukocyte count. These samples were collected from retro-orbital plexus of rats. Each sample was centrifuged at 500× g for 10 min at 4 °C; the cells in the pellet were washed in 0.5 mL saline, and total cells were counted using automated cell counter. In order to perform differential analyses, aliquots of the cells were placed onto slides and then stained with Field's stain to identify eosinophils, lymphocytes, or neutrophils using standard morphologic determinants.

2.7. Collection of Bronchoalveolar Lavage Fluid (BALF)

Ice-cold PBS (0.5 mL) was instilled into the lungs and BALF was obtained by three aspirations (total volume 1.5 mL) via tracheal cannulation [11]. Each BALF was centrifuged, and the supernatant collected was stored at 70 °C. Total inflammatory cell numbers were assessed by counting cells in at least five squares of a hemocytometer, after exclusion of dead cells stained with trypan blue. Cell pellets were suspended in 0.5 mL PBS, and 100 mL of each solution was spun onto a slide.

2.8. Lung Tissue Homogenate Preparation

After collection of BAL fluid, animals were sacrificed. About 1 g of the lung tissue was homogenized in buffer solution (2 mL) of phosphate-buffered saline in a ratio of 1:2 (w/v; 1 g tissue with 2 mL PBS, pH 7.4). Homogenates were centrifuged at 10,000× g for 15 min at 4 °C in a refrigerated centrifuge (Eltrec, India). The supernatants were divided into aliquots, then stored at 20 °C, and used for further evaluation [12].

2.9. Determination of Inflammatory Cytokines Using Enzyme-Linked Immunosorbent Assay (ELISA)

To determine the levels of cytokines in vivo, BALF and lung homogenate samples were collected 24 h after the final OVA challenge. IL-4, IL-13, IL-1 β and Tumor necrosis factor-alpha (TNF-α) were assayed with commercially available ELISA kits (Krishgen Biosystems, India).

2.10. Biochemical Estimation (Total Protein and Albumin)

The activity of albumin in serum, BAL and lungs were measured using commercially available reagent kits (ERBA Diagnostics, India). Blood was centrifuged at 6000 rpm for 10 min. Serum samples were collected and frozen at −80 °C until the time of analysis.

2.11. Enzyme-Linked Immunosorbent Assay (ELISA)

To determine the levels of cytokines in vivo, BALF and lung homogenate, samples were collected 24 h after the final OVA challenge. IL-4, IL-13, IL-1 β and Tumor necrosis factor-alpha (TNF-α) were assayed with commercially available ELISA kits (Krishgen Biosystems, India), according to the manufacturer's instruction.

2.12. Histopathological Examination

At the end of the study rats from each group were sacrificed by urethane and their lungs were excised, washed and cleaned with 0.9% saline and kept in 10% neutral formalin and given for histopathological examination by staining it with Haematoxylin and Eosin (H & E) [12]. These tissues were trimmed and routinely processed. Tissue processing was done to dehydrate in ascending grades of alcohol, clearing in xylene and embedded in paraffin wax. Paraffin wax embedded tissue blocks were sections at 4–5 μm thickness with the Rotary Microtome. All the slides were stained with Haematoxylin & Eosin (H & E) stain. The prepared slides were examined under microscope and photomicrographs were taken at 40×.

2.13. Statistical Analysis

The statistical evaluation was performed with the assistance of GraphPad prism 5 for 64 bit Windows Version. All the experimental groups were compared to assess the statistical significance using One-way analysis of variance (ANOVA). Each test was followed by the Dunnet's multiple comparison. The data are represented as mean ± SEM values and p values < 0.05 were considered as statistically significant.

3. Results

3.1. Effect of Treatment Combination on OVA Induced Alterations in Body Weight and Relative Lungs Weight

In the present study, negative control group were observed with reduced body weight and an increased relative lungs weight as compared to normal control group (** $p < 0.01$). However, Standard group showed significant reduction in body weight as compared to normal control (** $p < 0.01$). Combination 2 group restored the decrease in body weight as compared to negative control (## $p < 0.01$) (Table 1)

Table 1. Effect of treatment combination on OVA induced alterations in Body Weight and Relative lungs weight.

Parameter	Normal Control	Negative Control	Standard	Combination 1	Combination 2
Body weight (gm)	273 ± 4.74	202 ± 3.94 **	193 ± 3.16 **	210.2 ± 3.26 **	223.2 ± 4.79 **##
Relative Lungs weight (gm)	0.72 ± 4.55	1.76 ± 0.20 **	0.87 ± 1.47	1.02 ± 2.14 **	0.95 ± 3.17 *

Data were analyzed by one-way ANOVA followed by Dunnett's Multiple Comparisons Test. Values are expressed as Mean ± S.E.M. (n = 6). Statistical significance was assessed as * $p < 0.05$, ** $p < 0.01$ vs normal control group and ## $p < 0.01$ vs. negative control group. Standard: 0.1 mg/kg dexamethasone + 0.5 mg/kg salbutamol, Combination 1: 30 mg/kg CSE + 0.5 mg/kg salbutamol, Combination 2: 60 mg/kg CSE + 0.5 mg/kg salbutamol.

3.2. Effect of Treatment Combination on OVA-Induced Alteration in Hematological Parameters

Evaluation of different hematological parameters provides better understanding of the diseased state. In the present study, significant changes in hematological parameters of negative control rats were observed as compared to normal control rats. As compared to normal control group, a significant decrease in hemoglobin, red blood cells (RBC) count, PCV%, MCV% was observed, in negative control group (** $p < 0.01$). Treatment combinations (30 mg/kg CSE + 0.5 mg/kg salbutamol, 60mg/kg CSE + 0.5 mg/kg salbutamol) significantly ameliorated these alterations observed in hematological parameters as compared to negative control rats (## $p < 0.01$). Standard combination (0.1 mg/kg dexamethasone + 0.5 mg/kg salbutamol) also decreased these aforementioned hematological parameters as compared to negative control group (## $p < 0.01$). In case of mean platelet count, WBCs, neutrophils and lymphocytes, a significant increase was observed in negative control group as compared to normal control group (** $p < 0.01$). When compared with normal control rats, Treatment combinations (30 mg/kg CSE + 0.5 mg/kg salbutamol, 60 mg/kg CSE + 0.5 mg/kg salbutamol) and standard group showed significant inhibition in differential WBCs, neutrophil and lymphocyte count (## $p < 0.01$). (Table 2)

Table 2. Effect of treatment combination on OVA-induced alteration in hematological parameters and differential cell counts in BAL fluid of rats.

Parameter	Normal Control	Negative Control	Standard	Treatment 1	Treatment 2
Hemoglobin (gm/dl)	15.05 ± 0.25	11.15 ± 0.11 **	14.38 ± 0.35 **##	12.73 ± 0.11 **##	13.93 ± 0.24 **##
RBC	8.84 ± 0.2	8.18 ± 0.12	8.74 ± 0.10	8.09 ± 0.16	8.76 ± 0.23
PCV%	43.2 ± 1.34	35.98 ± 0.86 **	44.11 ± 0.83 ##	37.73 ± 0.43 **	41.91 ± 1.51 ##
MCV%	47.93 ± 0.42	41.05 ± 0.34 **	48.78 ± 1.44 ##	46.03 ± 1.20 ##	46.88 ± 0.78 ##
Mean Platelets	4.84 ± 0.30	8.24 ± 0.67 ***	5.46 ± 0.19 ##	7.10 ± 0.69 *	6.01 ± 0.35 #
WBC ($\times 10^3/mm^3$)	15.83 ± 0.85	26.89 ± 1.49 **	16.41 ± 0.56 ##	19.88 ± 1.30 *##	18.45 ± 1.13 ##
N (%)	28.5 ± 1.05	46.16 ± 1.03 **	29.83 ± 0.87 ##	35.5 ± 0.42 **##	66 ± 0.89 ##
L (%)	62.83 ± 1.40	74.33 ± 1.41 **	63.66 ± 1.28 ##	32.66 ± 0.76 *##	64.83 ± 0.98 ##
BALF-Total cell count	9.63 ± 0.52	49.85 ± 2.53 ***	15.01 ± 1.05	27.45 ± 1.24 ***	21.09 ± 1.79 ***
N ($\times 10^3$)	2.69 ± 0.17	15.32 ± 1.66 **	4.17 ± 0.28 ##	8.35 ± 0.42 *##	6.18 ± 0.54 **##
L ($\times 10^3$)	3.113 ± 0.23	15.57 ± 1.62 **	4.72 ± 0.33 ##	9.33 ± 0.42 **##	7.80 ± 0.76 **##
E ($\times 10^3$)	0.16 ± 0.02	2.29 ± 0.22 **	0.22 ± 0.04 ##	0.77 ± 0.04 **##	0.67 ± 0.09 *##
M ($\times 10^3$)	0.15 ± 0.17	1.39 ± 0.19 **	0.26 ± 0.02 ##	1.09 ± 0.04 **	0.53 ± 0.10 *##
Epithelial cells ($\times 10^3$)	3.507 ± 0.21	15.26 ± 0.51 **	5.45 ± 0.42 ##	7.89 ± 0.52 **##	5.89 ± 0.50 ##

Data were analyzed by one-way ANOVA followed by Dunnett's Multiple Comparisons Test. Values are expressed as Mean ± S.E.M. (n = 6). Statistical significance was assessed as * $p < 0.05$, ** $p < 0.01$, *** $p < 0.001$ vs. normal control group and # $p < 0.05$, ## $p < 0.01$, vs. negative control group. N—Neutrophils, L—Lymphocytes, E—Eosinophils, M—Monocytes. Standard: 0.1 mg/kg dexamethasone + 0.5 mg/kg salbutamol, Combination 1: 30 mg/kg CSE + 0.5 mg/kg salbutamol, Combination 2: 60 mg/kg CSE + 0.5 mg/kg salbutamol.

3.3. Inflammatory and Differential Cell Counts in BALF

BALF differential and total cell counts were increased significantly in negative control rats as compared to normal control (*** $p < 0.001$). However, Treatment combination groups (30 mg/kg CSE + 0.5 mg/kg salbutamol, 60mg/kg CSE + 0.5 mg/kg salbutamol) showed significant decrease in BAL fluid count as compared to negative control group (### $p < 0.001$). Also in case of Standard (0.1 mg/kg dexamethasone + 0.5 mg/kg salbutamol) group BALF total and differential cell count were significantly decreased as compared to negative control group (## $p < 0.01$)

3.4. Effect of Treatment Combination on OVA-Induced Alteration in the Levels of Total Protein in Serum, BALF and Lung Tissues of Rats

In the present investigation, Negative control rats showed significant increase in total protein levels in serum (** $p < 0.01$), BALF (** $p < 0.01$) and lung tissues (** $p < 0.01$) as compared to normal control rats. Increase in total protein and albumin was significantly inhibited by treatment combinations (30 mg/kg CSE+ 0.5 mg/kg salbutamol, 60 mg/kg CSE + 0.5 mg/kg salbutamol) in serum, BALF and lung tissues (## p < 0.01) as compared to negative control rats. Standard group (0.1 mg/kg dexamethasone + 0.5 mg/kg salbutamol) significantly decreased total protein levels in serum, BALF and lung tissues of rats (## p < 0.01) as compared to negative control group.

3.5. Effect of Treatment Combination on OVA-Induced Alteration in Albumin Levels in Serum and BALF

An increase in albumin levels in serum and BALF of negative control group was observed as compared to normal control group (** p < 0.01). However standard group (0.1 mg/kg dexamethasone + 0.5 mg/kg salbutamol) and treatment groups (30 mg/kg CSE + 0.5 mg/kg salbutamol, 60 mg/kg CSE + 0.5 mg/kg salbutamol) decreased albumin levels in serum and BALF (## p < 0.01) as compared to negative control group. (Refer Table 3)

Table 3. Effect of treatment combination on OVA-induced alteration in the levels of total protein and albumin in serum, BALF and lung tissues of rats.

Parameter	Normal Control	Negative Control	Standard	Combination 1	Combination 2
Serum total protein (gm/dl)	7.36 ± 0.20	9.43 ± 0.21 **	7.66 ± 0.20 ##	9.43 ± 0.21 **	8.36 ± 0.20 *#
BALF total protein (gm/dl)	1.12 ± 0.06	2.98 ± 0.04 **	1.27 ± 0.05 ##	1.95 ± 0.08 **##	1.52 ± 0.07 *##
Lung total protein (gm/dl)	0.822 ± 0.11	2.26 ± 0.08 **	1.17 ± 0.03 *##	1.37 ± 0.10 **##	1.83 ± 0.05 *##
Serum albumin (gm/dl)	0.56 ± 0.02	1.11 ± 0.04 **	0.59 ± 0.05 ##	0.89 ± 0.07 **#	0.69 ± 0.08 ##
BALF albumin (gm/dl)	0.084 ± 0.02	0.17 ± 0.02 **	0.112 ± 0.01 #	0.11 ± 0.03 ##	0.098 ± 0.02 ##

Data were analyzed by one-way ANOVA followed by Dunnett's Multiple Comparisons Test. Values are expressed as Mean ± S.E.M. (n = 6). Statistical significance was assessed as * p < 0.05, ** p < 0.01 vs. normal control group and # p < 0.05, ## p < 0.01 vs. negative control group. Standard: 0.1 mg/kg dexamethasone + 0.5 mg/kg salbutamol, Combination 1: 30 mg/kg CSE+ 0.5 mg/kg salbutamol, Combination 2: 60 mg/kg CSE + 0.5 mg/kg salbutamol.

3.6. Effect of Treatment Combination on OVA-Induced Alteration in Cytokine Analysis of BALF and Lung Tissues

Higher levels of Th2 response related cytokines (TNF-α and IL's) shows successful induction of asthma. In the current study, a significant up-regulation was observed in cytokine levels (IL-4, IL-13, IL-1 β, TNF-α) (** p < 0.01) of negative control group as compared to normal control group in both lung tissue and BALF. In case of IL-4, combination 2 group showed significant reduction in IL-4 levels as compared to negative control group in lung tissues and BALF of normal control (* p < 0.05) and negative control group (## p < 0.01) respectively. Up-regulation of IL-13 levels were inhibited by standard and treatment groups in lung tissues and BALF as compared to negative control group (## p < 0.01). IL-1β levels in lung tissue of standard and treatment groups were significantly reduced as compared to negative control group (## p < 0.01). Levels of TNF-α was reduced in both standard and treatment groups as compared to negative control group (## p < 0.01). (Figure 2)

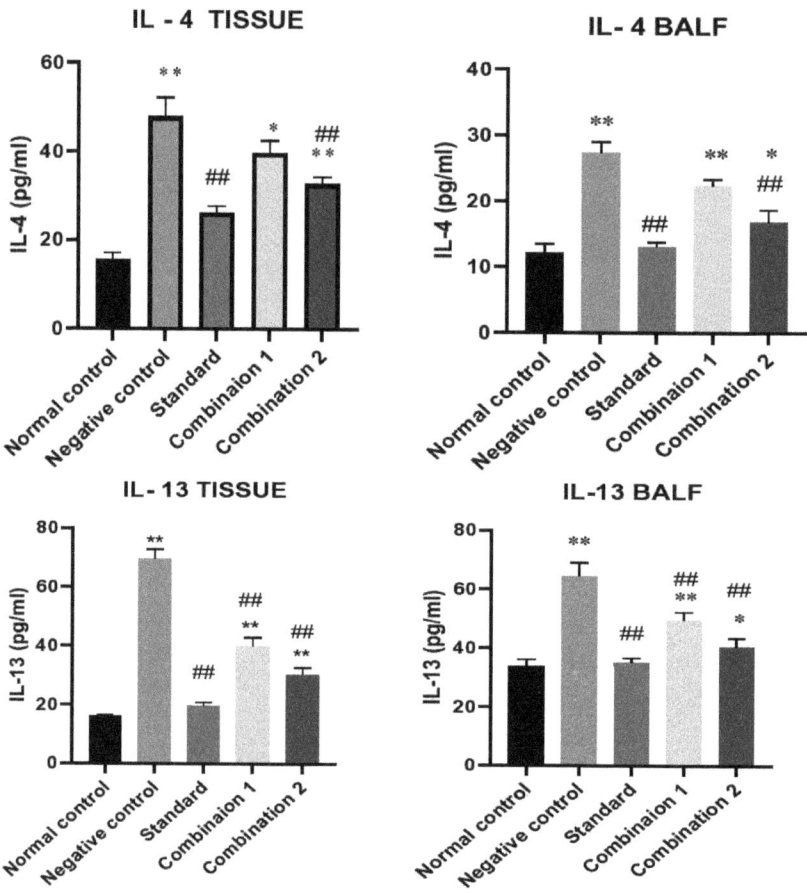
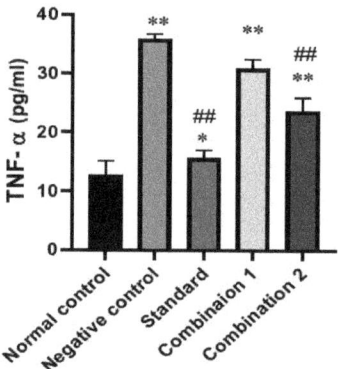

Figure 2. *Cont.*

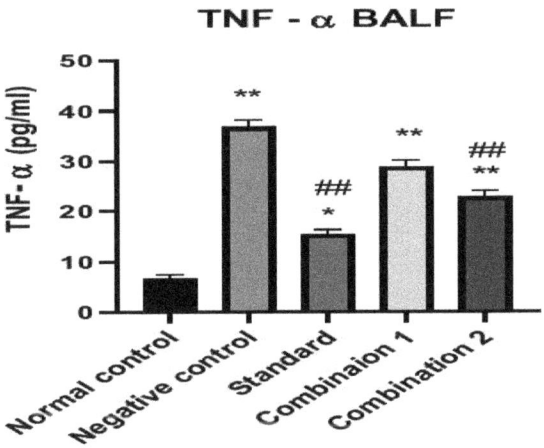

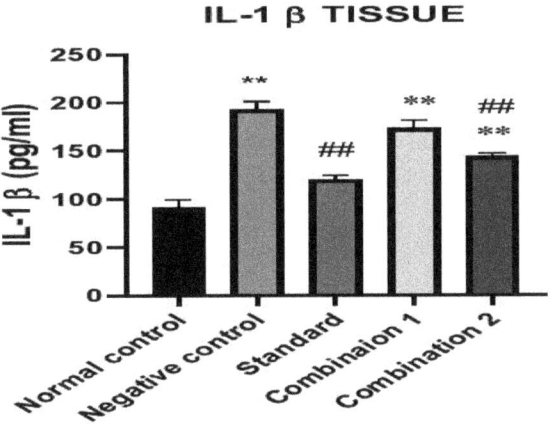

Figure 2. Effect of treatment combination on OVA-induced alteration in Cytokine analysis (IL-4, IL-13, TNF-α, IL-1β) of lung tissues and BALF. Data were analyzed by one-way ANOVA followed by Dunnett's Multiple Comparisons Test. Values are expressed as Mean ± S.E.M. (n = 4). Statistical significance was assessed as * $p < 0.05$, ** $p < 0.01$ vs. normal control group and # $p < 0.05$, ## $p < 0.01$ vs. negative control group. Standard: 0.1 mg/kg dexamethasone + 0.5 mg/kg salbutamol, Combination 1: 30 mg/kg CSE + 0.5 mg/kg salbutamol, Combination 2: 60 mg/kg CSE + 0.5 mg/kg salbutamol.

3.7. Effect of Treatment Combination on OVA-Induced Histopathological Alteration in Rat Lungs

The following pathological changes were observed in the lungs: interstitial infiltration (eosinophil and lymphocyte), grade of infiltration and other notable changes. Normal control group showed no leukocyte or eosinophil infiltration and no notable changes in the lung tissues were observed. However, in the case of the negative control group, mild eosinophilic infiltrations were observed followed by moderate to severe leukocytic infiltration. A minimal degree of hemorrhage was also observed. Standard group showed minimal leukocytic infiltration. As in the case of treatment groups, minimal eosinophilic infiltration was observed and mild to moderate leukocytic infiltrations were observed. However, treatment groups, like negative control group, also showed minimum degree of hemorrhage (Table 4) (Figure 3). Following were the levels of observed grade of infiltration for each group.

Table 4. Histopathological findings.

Groups	Eosinophilic Infiltration	Leukocyte Infiltration	Other Changes	Grade of Infiltration
Normal control	Not noted	Not noted	Not noted	00
Negative control	Mild	Moderate to severe	Minimal degree hemorrhage	3–4
Standard	—	Minimal	—	0–1
Combination 1	Minimal	Mild to moderate	Minimal degree hemorrhage	2
Combination 2	Minimal	Mild	Minimal degree hemorrhage	1–2

Standard: 0.1 mg/kg dexamethasone + 0.5 mg/kg salbutamol, Combination 1: 30 mg/kg CSE + 0.5 mg/kg salbutamol, Combination 2: 60 mg/kg CSE+ 0.5 mg/kg salbutamol.

Photomicrograph of sections of lungs of:

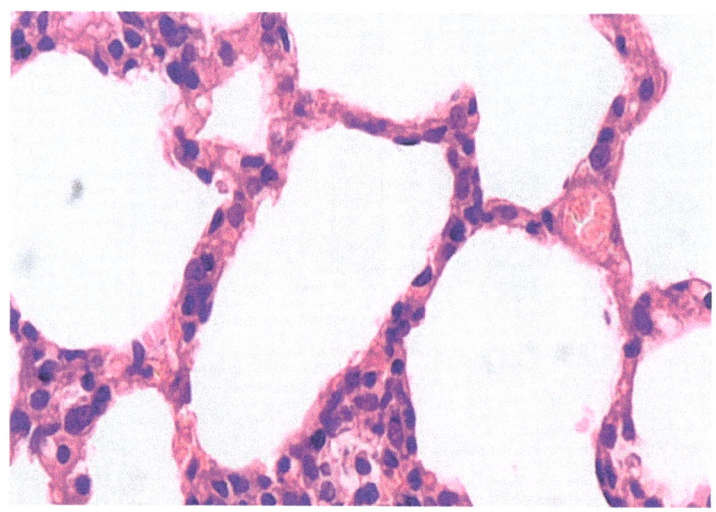

Normal Control:

- No hemorrhage noted

A **Normal Control:** No eosinophilic/ leukocytic infiltrations in the lungs were observed.

Figure 3. Cont.

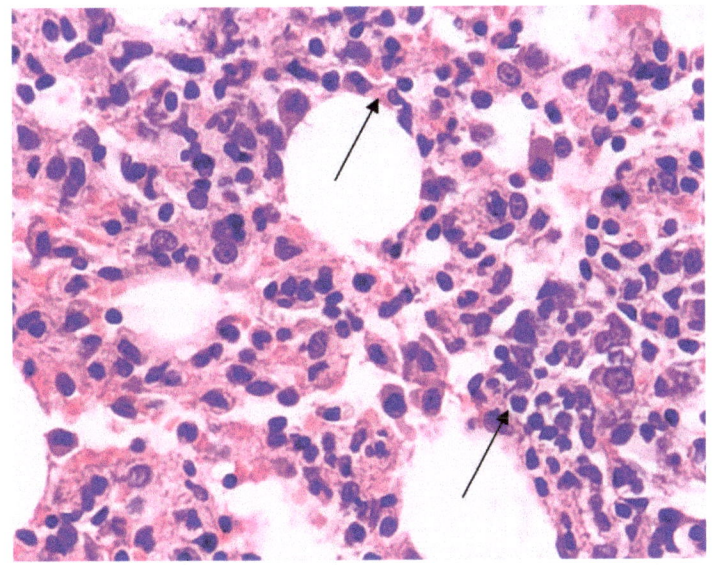

B Negative Control: Arrow indicates marked grade of eosinophilic & leukocyte infiltration in the lungs.

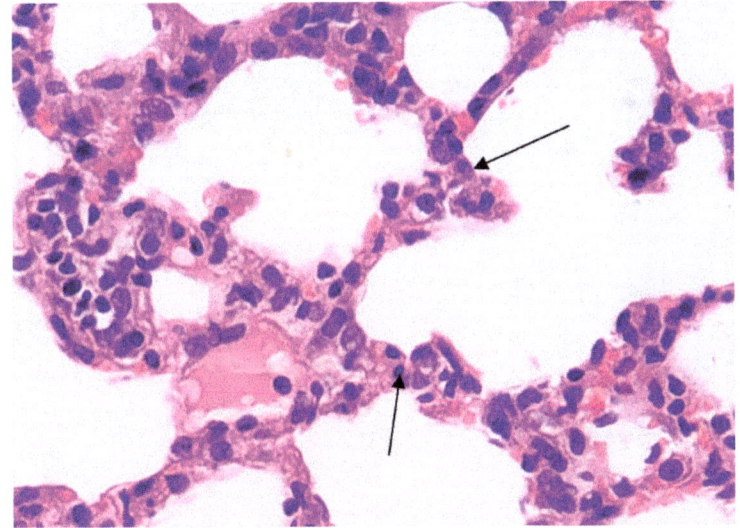

C Standard: Arrow indicates minimal grade of leukocytic infiltration in the lungs.

Figure 3. *Cont.*

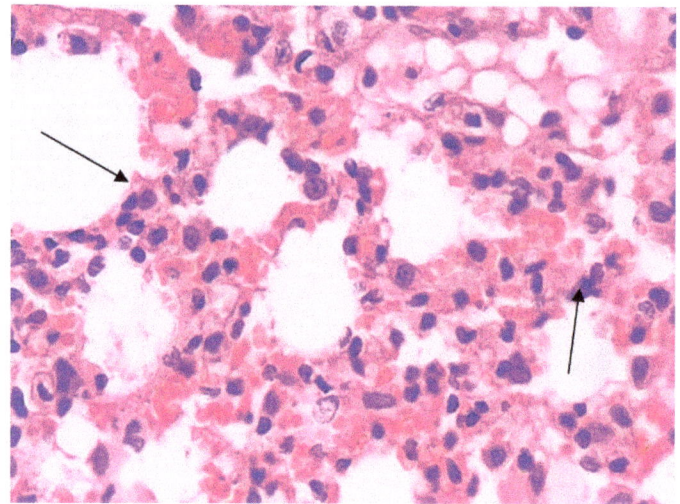

D Combination I: Arrow indicates minimal grade of eosinophilic infiltration in the lungs.

Combination I:

- Minimal eosinophilic infiltration
- Mild to moderate leukocyte infiltration

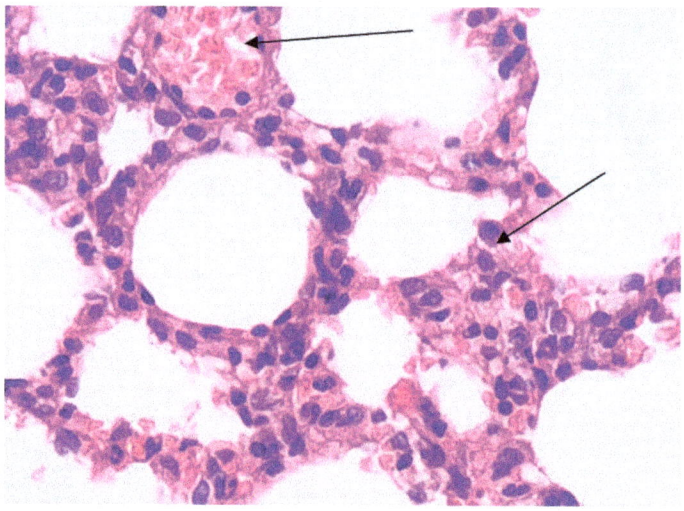

E Combination II: Arrow indicates minimal grade of eosinophilic & leukocyte infiltration in the lungs.

Combination II:

- Minimal eosinophilic infiltration
- Mild leukocyte infiltration
- Minimal degree

Figure 3. Effect of treatment combination on OVA-induced alteration in lung histology of rats.

4. Discussion

Asthma is a chronic, immunoinflammatory disorder of the airways characterized by airway hyperresponsiveness, mucus hypersecretion and bronchial inflammation. It is a well-known fact that asthma leads to chronic inflammation of the tracheo-bronchial tree [13]. Several animal models have given us insights about the probable mechanisms involved in the pathogenesis of asthma. In the present study, we have evaluated the combined effects of saffron extract (*C. sativus*) along with salbutamol, in OVA—induced model of asthma. Administration of saffron extract (*C. sativus*) and salbutamol in OVA—challenged rats increased body weights, improved hematological parameters. It inhibited infiltration of BALF cells, improved biochemical parameters (total protein and albumin). The combination also decreased inflammatory cytokine (IL-4, IL-13, TNF-α, IL-1β) levels and improved histopathological parameters of the lung tissue. Thus, these results show the anti-asthmatic activity of saffron extract—salbutamol in an OVA-challenged model of allergic airway inflammation.

A decrease in body weight of rats was observed in standard group as compared to negative control group. This could be attributed to the fact that, daily dose of dexamethasone reduced 5-HT (hydroxytryptamine) levels in the brain. Moreover, dexamethasone also elevated plasma leptin levels in a dose dependent manner [14,15]. Thus, cited literature suggests that leptin level in plasma may play a vital role in dexamethasone-induced anorexia. However, treatment combination groups showed significant improvement in body weights as compared to negative control group. Literature suggests that macrophages play a vital role in innate immune responses [16]. In an inflammatory state, lung tissue cells attract and infiltrate eosinophils, neutrophils, and lymphocytes from the blood. causing bronchial hyperresponsiveness. Thus, increase in the number of eosinophils is a prominent feature of allergic asthma leading to several inflammatory reactions. As a result, these inflammatory reactions play a detrimental role in causing damage to endothelial cells and extracellular matrix (ECM) present in the airways. In line with previous findings [17], results obtained from this study showed alterations in hematological differential cell counts, eosinophil and neutrophil counts, increase in total WBC counts in negative control group after OVA-challenge. Results from current investigation indicate improvement in hematological parameters after administration of saffron extract—salbutamol. Similarly, results obtained from total and differential cell count in BAL fluid of negative control group showed significant aberrations as compared to normal control group, whereas administration of treatment combination inhibited it. Shredding of epithelial cells occurs in the airways and is considered as a hallmark in airway inflammation. The present study also shows increase in epithelial shredding of the airways in negative control group as compared to normal control group. Treatment combination inhibited it to a certain extent.

Increase in protein and albumin levels are considered as a characteristic feature of tissue damage. Thus, the effect of treatment combination on total protein (TP) and albumin levels were studied. Reports from the present study indicate that treatment of OVA sensitized animals with saffron extract and salbutamol prevented increase in TP levels. However, a significant increase in TP levels of negative control group was observed in serum, BALF and lung tissues as compared to normal control group. These results are in line with previous research findings [18]. Similarly, from the present investigation BALF and serum albumin reports suggest that treatment combination has significantly inhibited albumin levels in OVA sensitized rats.

It is well documented that pathogenesis of asthma is due to infiltration of Th2 cytokines (IL-4, IL-13) and they also play an important role in the inflammatory mechanism of allergic asthma [19]. Switching of B lymphocyte to produce IgE and activation of macrophage and dendritic cells requires signals by Th2 cells, mainly IL-4. IL-13 activates signal transducer and transcription factor (STAT 6) via IL-4 mediated signal transduction, leading to AHR in the allergic lung [20,21]. Thus, Th2 cytokines play a significant role in regulating allergic responses. In this study, it was observed that IL-4 and IL-13 levels in lung tissues and BALF were significantly increased in negative control group. Results reveal that administration of saffron extract and salbutamol inhibited the levels of Th2 cytokines, IL-4 and IL-13 in both BALF and lung tissues.

TNF-α and IL-1β are pleiotropic cytokines which drive inflammatory responses causing changes in airway smooth muscle (ASM) responsiveness in asthma. Asthmatics have demonstrated high levels of these pro-inflammatory cytokines in the BAL fluid which are responsible for contraction of ASM [22]. Taking these evidences into consideration, levels of TNF-α and IL-1β in rat lung tissues and BALF were studied. In negative control rats, an upregulation of TNF- α and IL-1β levels were observed after OVA challenge. However, treatment combination inhibited this pro-inflammatory mediator, thus showing its anti-inflammatory effect. Data from the present study indicate that treatment combination of saffron extract and salbutamol decreased the levels of TNF-α and IL-1β in lung tissue as compared to negative control group, thus showing its anti-inflammatory potential against allergen-induced immunoinflammatory disease. The finding of the previous investigator [23] also showed the anti- inflammatory potential of saffron extract via inhibition of TNF-α and IL-1β and our results are also in line with the findings of the investigator.

Inflammatory infiltration in the lungs due to tissue damage is a unique histological feature of OVA challenged allergic asthma model. Histopathological findings illustrated moderate to severe eosinophilic and leukocytic infiltrations along with minimal hemorrhage in the lung tissues of OVA exposed rats of negative control group. However, saffron extract and salbutamol treated rats showed minimal degree of inflammatory infiltration along with minimal hemorrhage in the lungs. Thus, this treatment combination ameliorated histological aberrations caused by OVA inhalation.

5. Conclusions

Currently available treatment regimens for asthma focus on controlling asthmatic exacerbations and are associated with many side effects. Based upon the results obtained from the present study, the combination of *C. sativus* extract and salbutamol exhibits its anti-asthmatic activity against OVA induced allergic asthma. The treatment combination decreased total and differential cell count in blood and BALF, thereby showing its anti-inflammatory property. The treatment combination also ameliorated total protein, albumin levels, Th2 cytokines (IL-4 and IL-13) and immune-inflammatory responses (TNF-α and IL-1β) in lung tissues and BALF, thus exhibiting its immunomodulatory property. These results suggest that, combined effects of *C. sativus* extract and salbutamol can be considered as an "add-on therapy" for asthmatics or could be used along with current available anti-asthmatic drugs.

Author Contributions: Conceptualization K.P. and P.N. ; methodology, K.P. and P.N.; software, K.P. and P.N., validation, K.P., formal analysis, K.P., investigation, K.P. and P.N., resources, K.P. and P.N., data curation, K.P. and P.N., writing—original draft preparation, P.N., writing—P.N., visualization, K.P. and P.N., supervision, K.P., project administration, funding acquisition, N/A. All authors have read and agreed to the published version of the manuscript.

Funding: This research received no external funding.

Institutional Review Board Statement: The entire experimental protocol was reviewed and approved by an Institutional Animal Ethics Committee registered under "Committee for the Purpose of Control and Supervision of Experiment on Laboratory Animals" (CPCSEA), Ministry of Environment and Forests, Government of India. Approval number—CPCSEA/IAEC/P-34/2018.

Informed Consent Statement: Not applicable.

Data Availability Statement: The data presented in this study are available on request from the corresponding author.

Conflicts of Interest: The authors declare no conflict of interest.

References

1. Symptoms, R. Economic burden of asthma in India. *Lung India Off. Organ Indian Chest Soc.* **2018**, *35*, 281.
2. Nakagome, K.; Matsushita, S.; Nagata, M. Neutrophilic inflammation in severe asthma. *Int. Arch. Allergy Immunol.* **2012**, *158*, 96–102. [CrossRef] [PubMed]
3. Calhoun, W.J. Nocturnal Asthma. *Chest* **2003**, *123*, 399–405. [CrossRef] [PubMed]
4. Access, O.; Keglowich, L.F.; Borger, P. The Three A's in Asthma—Airway Smooth Muscle. *Airw. Remodel. Angiogenesis* **2015**, 70–80. [CrossRef]
5. Barnes, P. Drugs for asthma. *Br. J. Pharmacol.* **2016**, *147*, S297–S303. [CrossRef]

6. Tal, A.; Bavilski, C.; Yohai, D.; Bearman, J.E.; Gorodischer, R.; Moses, S.W. Dexamethasone and salbutamol in the treatment of acute wheezing in infants. *Pediatrics* **1983**, *71*, 13–18.
7. Pauwels, R.A.; Löfdahl, C.G.; Postma, D.S.; Tattersfield, A.E.; O'Byrne, P.; Barnes, P.J.; Ullman, A. Effect of inhaled formoterol and budesonide on exacerbations of asthma. Formoterol and Corticosteroids Establishing Therapy (FACET) International Study Group. *N. Engl. J. Med.* **1997**, *337*, 1405–1411, Erratum in: *N. Engl. J. Med.* **1998**, *338*, 139. [CrossRef]
8. Plint, A.C.; Johnson, D.W.; Patel, H.; Wiebe, N.; Correll, R.; Brant, R.; Mitton, C.; Gouin, S.; Bhatt, M.; Joubert, G.; et al. Pediatric Emergency Research Canada (PERC). Epinephrine and dexamethasone in children with bronchiolitis. *N. Engl. J. Med.* **2009**, *360*, 2079–2089. [CrossRef]
9. Pitsikas, N.; Sakellaridis, N. Crocus sativus L. extracts antagonize memory impairments in different behavioural tasks in the rat. *Behav. Brain Res.* **2006**, *173*, 112–115. [CrossRef]
10. Salami, E.O.; Ozolua, R.I.; Okpo, S.O.; Eze, G.I.; Uwaya, D.O. Studies on the anti—Asthmatic and antitussive properties of aqueous leaf extract of Bryophyllum pinnatum in rodent species. *Asian Pac. J. Trop. Med.* **2013**, *6*, 421–425. [CrossRef]
11. Mukherjee, A.A.; Kandhare, A.D.; Rojatkar, S.R.; Bodhankar, S.L. Ameliorative effects of Artemisia pallens in a murine model of ovalbumin-induced allergic asthma via modulation of biochemical perturbations. *Biomed. Pharmacother.* **2017**, *94*, 880–889. [CrossRef] [PubMed]
12. Zemmouri, H.; Sekiou, O.; Ammar, S.; El Feki, A.; Bouaziz, M.; Messarah, M.; Boumendjel, A. Urtica dioica attenuates ovalbumin-induced inflammation and lipid peroxidation of lung tissues in rat asthma model. *Pharm. Biol.* **2017**, *55*, 1561–1568. [CrossRef] [PubMed]
13. Ye, W.-J.; Xu, W.-G.; Guo, X.-J.; Han, F.-F.; Peng, J.; Li, X.-M.; Guan, W.-B.; Yu, L.-W.; Sun, J.-Y.; Cui, Z.-L.; et al. Differences in airway remodeling and airway inflammation among moderate-severe asthma clinical phenotypes. *J. Thorac. Dis.* **2017**, *9*, 2904–2914. [CrossRef] [PubMed]
14. Jahng, J.W.; Kim, N.Y.; Ryu, V.; Yoo, S.B.; Kim, B.T.; Kang, D.W.; Lee, J.H. Dexamethasone reduces food intake, weight gain and the hypothalamic 5-HT concentration and increases plasma leptin in rats. *Eur. J. Pharmacol.* **2008**, *581*, 64–70. [CrossRef] [PubMed]
15. Michel, C.; Cabanac, M. Effects of dexamethasone on the body weight set point of rats. *Physiol. Behav.* **1999**, *68*, 145–150. [CrossRef]
16. Parihar, A.; Eubank, D.; Doseff, A.I. Monocytes and Macrophages Regulate Immunity through Dynamic Networks of Survival and Cell Death. *J. Innate Immun.* **2010**, *43220*, 204–215. [CrossRef]
17. Vosooghi, S.; Mahmoudabady, M.; Neamati, A.; Aghababa, H. Preventive effects of hydroalcoholic extract of saffron on hematological parameters of experimental asthmatic rats. *Avicenna J. Phytomed.* **2013**, *3*, 279–27987.
18. Gholamnezhad, Z.; Koushyar, H.; Byrami, G.; Boskabady, M.H. The Extract of Crocus sativus and Its Constituent Safranal, Affect Serum Levels of Endothelin and Total Protein in Sensitized Guinea Pigs. *Iran J Basic Med Sci* **2013**, *16*, 1022–1026.
19. Palmqvist, C.; Wardlaw, A.J.; Bradding, P. Chemokines and their receptors as potential targets for the treatment of asthma. *Br. J. Pharmacol.* **2007**, *151*, 725–736. [CrossRef]
20. Poulsen, L.K.; Hummelshoj, L. Triggers of IgE class switching and allergy development. *Ann. Med.* **2007**, *39*, 440–456. [CrossRef]
21. Muraro, A.; Lemanske, R.F.; Hellings, P.W.; Akdis, C.A.; Bieber, T.; Casale, T.B.; Jutel, M.; Ong, P.Y.; Poulsen, L.K.; Schmid-Grendelmeier, P.; et al. Precision medicine in patients with allergic diseases: Airway diseases and atopic dermatitis—PRACTALL document of the European Academy of Allergy and Clinical Immunology and the American Academy of Allergy, Asthma & Immunology. *J. Allergy Clin. Immunol.* **2016**, *137*, 1347–1358. [CrossRef] [PubMed]
22. Dejager, L.; Dendoncker, K.; Eggermont, M.; Souffriau, J.; Van Hauwermeiren, F.; Willart, M.; Van Wonterghem, E.; Naessens, T.; Ballegeer, M.; Vandevyver, S.; et al. Neutralizing TNFα restores glucocorticoid sensitivity in a mouse model of neutrophilic airway inflammation. *Mucosal Immunol.* **2015**, *8*, 1212–1225. [CrossRef] [PubMed]
23. Xiong, Y.; Wang, J.; Yu, H.; Zhang, X.; Miao, C. Nti-asthma potential of crocin and its effect on MAPK signaling pathway in a murine model of allergic airway disease. *Immunopharmacol. Immunotoxicol.* **2015**, *37*, 236–243. [CrossRef] [PubMed]

Case Report

Low-Grade B Cell Lymphoproliferative Disorder Masquerading as Chronic Rhinosinusitis

Rory Chan *, Chris RuiWen Kuo and Brian Lipworth

Scottish Centre for Respiratory Research and Rhinology Mega-Clinic, School of Medicine, University of Dundee, Ninewells Hospital, Dundee DD1 9SY, UK; r.kuo@dundee.ac.uk (C.R.K.); b.j.lipworth@dundee.ac.uk (B.L.)
* Correspondence: rchan@dundee.ac.uk

Abstract: Chronic rhinosinusitis (CRS) is one of the most common persistent disorders of the developed world, requiring input from various specialists including primary care physicians, otolaryngologists, respiratory physicians, and allergologists. B-cell lymphoproliferative disorders (BLPDs) are a heterogenous group of malignant conditions defined by an accumulation of mature B lymphocytes in the bone marrow, blood, and lymphoid tissues. We present a case report of an elderly man with rhinosinusitis-like symptoms and atypical features prompting further investigations that culminated in a diagnosis of BLPD.

Keywords: chronic rhinosinusitis; B-cell lymphoproliferative disorder

1. Introduction

Chronic rhinosinusitis (CRS) is one of the most common persistent disorders of the developed world, requiring input from various specialists including primary care physicians, otolaryngologists, respiratory physicians, and allergologists [1]. Current international guidelines recommend that diagnosis is made by clinicians on the basis of symptoms such as nasal blockage, discharge, facial pressure, and loss of smell for at least 12 weeks [2]. However, the diagnostic work up can be fraught with difficulty, especially when attempting to differentiate between CRS and allergic and nonallergic rhinitis on symptoms alone. Additionally, not all patients with CRS criteria will have evidence of disease on nasal endoscopy and CT imaging [2].

Based on high quality evidence, medical therapy with long term nasal corticosteroids, short courses of oral corticosteroids, and/or nasal irrigation with isotonic saline or Ringer's lactate are effective in treating CRS [2]. Dupilumab (anti-IL4rα) is the only monoclonal antibody approved for the treatment of CRS with nasal polyps (CRSwNP) at present. Two studies have demonstrated efficacy of intravenous mepolizumab (anti-IL5) 750 mg q4w on reducing the need for nasal polyp surgery and total polyp score [3,4] but at the current subcutaneous licensed dose of 100 mg q4w, our experience has shown a clear disconnect in response between severe eosinophilic asthma and CRSwNP [5]. Surgical management is usually indicated when CRSwNP is refractory to medical therapy [2].

B-cell lymphoproliferative disorders (BLPDs) are a heterogenous group of malignant haematological conditions with a significantly higher incidence in individuals with primary or secondary immunodeficiency [6]. Diagnosis is usually made on the basis of clinical features such as enlarged lymph nodes or splenomegaly and excess fatigue and/or apparent cytopenia and lymphocytosis on a full blood count [7]. Morphological examination demonstrating a lymphocytic increase or abnormality would prompt further immunophenotypic investigations. Multiparameter flow cytometry on peripheral blood or bone marrow is a rapid and efficient tool for the diagnosis of BLPDs [7].

2. Case

A 72-year-old man was referred by his general practitioner for chronic bilateral nasal congestion, worse at night, and purulent nasal secretions predominantly in the morning. In addition to multiple courses of antibiotics, he had previously tried fluticasone furoate, mometasone furoate, and beclomethasone dipropionate nasal sprays to no avail. He retained his sense of smell and denied post-nasal drip, sneezing, breathlessness, or cough. He had no history of excess fatigue, weight loss, or night sweats. His past medical history included essential hypertension for which he was taking perindopril 2 mg once daily (OD) and a previous cerebral infarction treated with clopidogrel 75 mg OD. He is an ex-smoker with no relevant family history.

Nasal endoscopy (30° oblique rigid Hopkins 3.0 mm) performed in our rhinology mega-clinic revealed an oedematous friable bleeding nasal mucosal surface with significant crusting but no polyps per se. Biopsy samples were taken from the middle turbinate and crusting was debrided. Nasal douching with saline/bicarbonate was recommended, and he was treated with concurrent azithromycin 500 mg OD and prednisolone 25 mg OD for 5 and 7 days, respectively, pending further results.

Initial laboratory results and subsequent lymphocyte surface marker analysis are presented in Table 1. Protein electrophoresis identified two monoclonal bands consistent with IgM lambda and kappa bands quantifiable at 10 g/L. CT sinus scan (Figure 1) revealed mucosal disease predominantly affecting the ethmoid bullae and ostiomeatal complex, with a Lund Mackay score of 12. Apart from minor basal atelectasis, chest X-ray was normal. Histopathology subsequently revealed chronic non-specific inflammatory changes with mixed microbial flora abundant in gram-positive cocci.

Table 1. Laboratory results and lymphocyte surface marker analysis.

White Blood Cells ($\times 10^9$/L)	9.8	Corr. Calcium (mmol/L)	2.44
Haemoglobin (g/L)	136	C-reactive protein (mg/L)	<4
Haematocrit (%)	41.3	Sodium (mmol/L)	141
Platelets ($\times 10^9$/L)	328	Potassium (mmol/L)	4.8
Neutrophils ($\times 10^9$/L)	5.4	Urea (mmol/L)	6.4
Lymphocytes ($\times 10^9$/L)	3.5	Creatinine (μmol/L)	86
Eosinophils ($\times 10^9$/L)	0.14	PR3/MPO antibodies	negative
Plasma viscosity (mPa.s)	1.99 ↑	CTD screen	negative
Total bilirubin (μmol/L)	5	RAST to ABCDH	negative
ALT (U/L)	25	RAST to grass	weakly positive
ALP (U/L)	110	Total IgE (kU/L)	89.5
Albumin (g/L)	36	IgG (g/L)	9.94 (NR 5.5–13)
Pneumococcal ab (mg/L)	52.64	IgA (g/L)	1 (NR 0.5–4)
		IgM (g/L)	10.2 ↑ (NR 0.5–2.5)
CD3 (%)	88.57 ↑	CD19 (%)	3.53
CD3 ($\times 10^6$/L)	2922 ↑	CD19 ($\times 10^6$/L)	116
CD4 (%)	32.94 ↑	NK cells (%)	6.88
CD4 ($\times 10^6$/L)	1087	NK cells ($\times 10^6$/L)	227
CD8 (%)	53.6 ↑	CD4/CD8 ratio	0.62 ↓
CD8 ($\times 10^6$/L)	1769 ↑		

A = aspergillus fumigatus; ALP = alkaline phosphatase; ALT = alanine aminotransferase; B = silver birch; C = cat dander; CD = cluster of differentiation; CTD = connective tissue disease; D = dog dander; H = house dust mite; MPO = myeloperoxidase; NK = natural killer; NR = normal range; PR3 = proteinase-3; RAST = radioallergosorbent testing for specific IgE. ↑ and ↓ denote values outside NR.

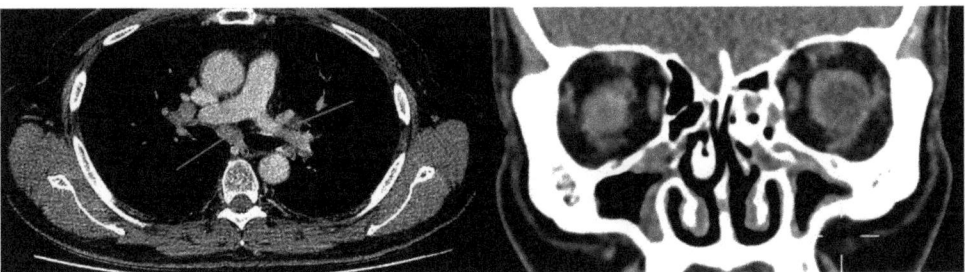

Figure 1. Transverse CT chest image with arrows indicating mediastinal and hilar lymphadenopathy. Coronal CT sinus image depicting disease affecting the ethmoid bullae and ostio-meatal complex.

Our patient was consequently referred to haematology where on physical examination there was no clinical evidence of palpable lymphadenopathy or hepatosplenomegaly. A CT chest-abdomen-pelvis scan (Figure 1) identified significant mediastinal and hilar lymphadenopathy and the combination of serum and radiological findings in turn made the clinical diagnosis of B-cell lymphoproliferative disorder (BLPD).

3. Discussion

In this case report, we present a patient referred from primary care for CRS without nasal polyposis and suspicious atypical features who was subsequently diagnosed with low grade BLPD. To our knowledge, although there have been case series on localised sinonasal lymphoma [8,9], we have not yet encountered a case report of BLPD masquerading as CRS.

While the diagnosis of BLPD was clinical, the value of endobronchial ultrasound-guided transbronchial needle aspiration (EBUS-TBNA) of mediastinal and hilar lymph nodes in the diagnosis of lymphoma is controversial [10] and hence a negative result would likely still mandate surgical mediastinoscopy confirmation. In the absence of B symptoms or abnormal full blood count, a watch and wait strategy is usually employed for low grade BLPDs and therefore no bone marrow or lymph nodes were sampled in our patient, to avoid unnecessary additional risk.

The abundance of gram-positive cocci is likely to infer chronic staphylococcal infection, which in turn is highly suggestive of immunosuppression. Although the acute abundance of gram-positive cocci commonly infers nasal colonisation with Streptococcus pneumoniae, failure to respond to recurrent courses of antibiotic therapy likely results in a selection pressure towards treatment resistant organisms such as Staphylococcus aureus [11]. Risk factors for S. aureus nasal colonisation depends on host factors but is more frequent in conditions that result in immunosuppression such as in patients infected with human immunodeficiency virus (HIV) or those who are diabetic and undergoing dialysis [12]. The combination of immunosuppression, IgM paraproteinaemia, and extensive mediastinal and hilar lymphadenopathy is probably sufficient to make a clinical diagnosis of BLPD.

The key learning point here is that although nasal crusting is a frequently encountered clinical feature that often requires no specific treatment, it is nevertheless crucial for the clinician to identify the small number of cases that are due to a potentially wide differential diagnosis including systemic inflammatory disorders such as vasculitis, malignancy, and infection, amongst others [13]. Clinicians should have a high index of clinical suspicion and our usual practice should be to check serum protein electrophoresis and immunoglobulins in all patients presenting with CRS-like symptoms and signs of immunosuppression as it may lead to an earlier diagnosis and potentially better outcome for patients.

4. Conclusions

Patients with chronic rhinosinusitis who present with atypical clinical features such as nasal crusting and treatment resistant organisms may have underlying immunosuppression. Identifying this in a timely manner with further focused investigations may lead to earlier diagnoses and better outcomes for patients.

Author Contributions: The manuscript has been read and approved by all the authors and the requirements for authorship have been met. We (authors) certify that we have (collectively) personally written 100 percent of the manuscript. The manuscript has not been published previously in print/electronic format or in another language and the manuscript is not under consideration by another publication or electronic media. All authors have read and agreed to the published version of the manuscript.

Funding: This research received no external funding.

Informed Consent Statement: Informed consent was obtained from all subjects involved in the study.

Data Availability Statement: Data sharing not applicable. No new data were created or analyzed in this study. Data sharing is not applicable to this article.

Conflicts of Interest: There are no financial conflict of interest to disclose.

References

1. Vaidyanathan, S.; Barnes, M.; Williamson, P.; Hopkinson, P.; Donnan, P.T.; Lipworth, B. Treatment of Chronic Rhinosinusitis With Nasal Polyposis With Oral Steroids Followed by Topical Steroids: A Randomized Trial. *Ann. Intern. Med.* **2011**, *154*, 293–302. [CrossRef] [PubMed]
2. Fokkens, W.J.; Lund, V.J.; Hopkins, C.; Hellings, P.W.; Kern, R.; Reitsma, S.; Toppila-Salmi, S.; Bernal-Sprekelsen, M.; Mullol, J.; Alobid, I.; et al. European Position Paper on Rhinosinusitis and Nasal Polyps 2020. *Rhinology* **2020**, *58*, 1–464. [CrossRef] [PubMed]
3. Bachert, C.; Sousa, A.R.; Lund, V.J.; Scadding, G.K.; Gevaert, P.; Nasser, S.; Durham, S.R.; Cornet, M.E.; Kariyawasam, H.H.; Gilbert, J.; et al. Reduced need for surgery in severe nasal polyposis with mepolizumab: Randomized trial. *J. Allergy Clin. Immunol.* **2017**, *140*, 1024–1031.e1014. [CrossRef] [PubMed]
4. Gevaert, P.; Van Bruaene, N.; Cattaert, T.; Van Steen, K.; Van Zele, T.; Acke, F.; De Ruyck, N.; Blomme, K.; Sousa, A.R.; Marshall, R.P.; et al. Mepolizumab, a humanized anti-IL-5 mAb, as a treatment option for severe nasal polyposis. *J. Allergy Clin. Immunol.* **2011**, *128*, 989–995. [CrossRef] [PubMed]
5. Chan, R.; Kuo, C.R.; Lipworth, B. Disconnect between effects of mepolizumab on severe eosinophilic asthma and chronic rhinosinusitis with nasal polyps. *J. Allergy Clin. Immunol.* **2020**. [CrossRef] [PubMed]
6. Knowles, D.M. Immunodeficiency-associated lymphoproliferative disorders. *Mod. Pathol.* **1999**, *12*, 200–217. [CrossRef] [PubMed]
7. Debord, C.; Wuillème, S.; Eveillard, M.; Theisen, O.; Godon, C.; Le Bris, Y.; Béné, M.C. Flow cytometry in the diagnosis of mature B-cell lymphoproliferative disorders. *Int. J. Lab. Hematol.* **2020**, *42*, 113–120. [CrossRef] [PubMed]
8. Steele, T.O.; Buniel, M.C.; Mace, J.C.; El Rassi, E.; Smith, T.L. Lymphoma of the nasal cavity and paranasal sinuses: A case series. *Am. J. Rhinol. Allergy* **2016**, *30*, 335–339. [CrossRef] [PubMed]
9. Peng, K.A.; Kita, A.E.; Suh, J.D.; Bhuta, S.M.; Wang, M.B. Sinonasal lymphoma: Case series and review of the literature. *Int. Forum Allergy Rhinol.* **2014**, *4*, 670–674. [CrossRef] [PubMed]
10. Erol, S.; Erer, O.F.; Anar, C.; Aktogu, S.; Aydogdu, Z. Diagnostic yield of EBUS-TBNA for mediastinal lymphoma. *Eur. Respir. J.* **2016**, *48*, PA3853. [CrossRef]
11. Brook, I. Microbiology of Sinusitis. *Proc. Am. Thorac. Soc.* **2011**, *8*, 90–100. [CrossRef] [PubMed]
12. Sakr, A.; Brégeon, F.; Mège, J.-L.; Rolain, J.-M.; Blin, O. Staphylococcus aureus Nasal Colonization: An Update on Mechanisms, Epidemiology, Risk Factors, and Subsequent Infections. *Front. Microbiol.* **2018**, *9*, 2419. [CrossRef] [PubMed]
13. Yaneza, M.M.; Broomfield, S.J.; Morar, P. 12 minute consultation: A patient with nasal crusting. *Clin. Otolaryngol.* **2010**, *35*, 313–320. [CrossRef] [PubMed]

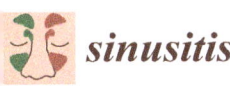 *sinusitis*

Article

Prevalence and Risk Factors of Sinus and Nasal Allergies among Tannery Workers of Kanpur City

Gyan Chandra Kashyap [1], Deepanjali Vishwakarma [2,*] and Shri Kant Singh [2]

1. Institute of Health Management Research, 319, Near Thimmareddy Layout, Hulimangala Post Electronic City Phase-1, Bangalore 560105, India; statskashyap@gmail.com
2. Department of Mathematical Demography & Statistics, International Institute for Population Sciences, Govandi Station Road, Deonar Mumbai 400088, India; sksingh1992@yahoo.co.in
* Correspondence: deepanjali.vishwakarma7@gmail.com

Abstract: India is greatly afflicted by sinusitis, which is a condition that involves inflaming sinuses (the air cavities in the nasal passage) in your nose, according to the National Institute of Allergy and Infectious Diseases (NIAID). The study's objective was to evaluate the prevalence and risk factors of sinus and nasal allergies among tannery workers of Kanpur city. The study has used primary datasets obtained from a cross-sectional household study of tannery workers from the Jajmau area of Kanpur in northern India, which was conducted during January–June 2015 as part of a doctoral program. The study covered 286 tannery workers from the study area. Bivariate and logistic regression analysis was used to study the association between outcome variables (self-reported prevalence of sinus and nasal allergies) and predictor variables (socioeconomic and work-related characteristics). Results portray that a higher proportion of the tannery workers belong to economically and socially backward classes. Overall, 13.4 and 12.3% of sinus and nasal allergy prevalence have been reported by tannery workers, whereas tannery workers from the oldest age group were those who mainly suffered. A study found that the severity of nasal and sinus allergies increases with the increasing age and work duration in the tannery. Workers with low exposure to airborne dust were significantly more likely to develop sinus problems (OR = 4.16; $p < 0.05$) than those without exposure. Those tannery workers suffering from nasal allergy were more prone to develop sinus problems than those who were not suffering from nasal allergy. The risk factors responsible for these health hazards can be eliminated by improving the overall working conditions and ensuring necessary protective regulations for the tannery workers.

Keywords: sinus; nasal allergies; tannery worker; Kanpur

1. Introduction

India is greatly afflicted by sinusitis, which is a condition that involves the inflaming of sinuses (the air cavities in the nasal passage) in your nose according to National Institute of Allergy and Infectious Diseases (NIAID). An estimated 134 million Indians suffer from chronic sinusitis, the symptoms of which include but are not limited to debilitating headaches, fever, and nasal congestion and obstruction [1]. Among Indians, this disease is more widespread than diabetes, asthma, or coronary heart disease. One in eight Indians suffer from chronic sinusitis caused by the inflammation of the nasal and throat lining, which results in the accumulation of mucus in the sinus cavity and pressure build-up in the face, eyes, and brain [2,3].

In the leather tanning process, during skin contact, chromium has the potential to bind with the skin proteins of the workers, producing complex antigen, which leads to hypersensitivity and dermatitis. Chromium leather in industries can cause carcinoma of the larynx and lung parenchyma and paranasal sinuses in workers [4–6]. In addition to these, scores of other chemicals and organic solvents such as chromate and bichromate salts, aniline, buty acetate, ethanol, benzene, toluene, sulfuric acid, and ammonium hydrogen sulfide are used in the tannery industry. An important health risk factor for the tannery workers is occupational exposure to chromium, mainly in the organic Cr (III) form or in the protein bound form (leather dust). Chromium may enter the body by inhalation, ingestion, and by direct cutaneous contact. Professional exposure to Cr (III) increases the risk of dermatitis, ulcers, and perforation of the nasal septum and respiratory illnesses as well as increased lung and nasal cancers. Work within the tannery itself is fraught with danger. When inhaled, chromium acts as a lung irritant and carcinogen, affecting the upper respiratory tract, obstructing airways, and increasing the chances of developing lung, nasal, or sinus cancer [7–14]. Limited studies have reported associations between occupational exposure, particularly the exposure of airborne dust and chemicals in the air, to tannery chemicals with sinus and nasal allergy among the tannery workers, and none have been conducted to study the occupational exposures with the sinus and nasal allergies in India. Even the most recent study based on tannery workers conducted in Bangladesh has not investigated the sinus and nasal allergy issue [15]. With this backdrop, this study has attempted to study the association between outcome variables (self-reported prevalence of sinus and nasal allergies) and predictor variables (socioeconomic and work-related characteristics). The specific objective was to estimate the prevalence and risk factors of Sinus and nasal allergies among tannery workers of Kanpur city, India.

2. Methods and Material

2.1. Data

A study has utilized the data from the cross-sectional household study of tannery and non-tannery workers from the Jajmau area of Kanpur. The study was conducted during January–June 2015, and all data were collected by the first author from the field. The first author of the study has interviewed 284 tannery and 289 non-tannery workers.

2.2. Study Area

The city Kanpur has conventionally been an industrial city and a major commercial center in Uttar Pradesh. There are currently 402 registered leather tanneries located in the eastern part of the city, with an estimated 20,000 tannery workers [7]. More than 20,000 people worked in the leather industry, and a substantial proportion of tannery workers were living in the Jajmau Area. From the significant concentrations of the tannery industry in and around Kanpur, Jajmau was selected for the study. It is known as the Leather City, as it contains some of the largest and finest tanneries in India. This study focused on leather tannery workers, i.e., those engaged in tanning work in the leather industry (Figure 1).

2.3. Sampling Design

A three-stage sampling design was used in this study. At the primary stage, seven localities in the Jajmau area, namely Tadbagiya, Kailash Nagar, J.K. colony, Asharfabad, Motinagar, Chabeelepurwa, and Budhiyaghat, were selected based on a higher concentration of leather tannery workers' households in these areas as informed by several stakeholders in the city. In the second stage, three out of the seven localities, namely Budhiyaghat, Tadbagiya, and Asharfabad, were chosen using the probability proportional to size (PPS) sampling technique after positioning them in growing order of assessed number of HHs of leather tannery workers. Afterward, an inclusive household listing and mapping was finished in each of the three localities. Moreover, all the listed households were classified into three groups: households having at least one tannery worker, irrespective of having any non-tannery worker, households with non-tannery worker(s), and households having no workers.

The first two groups were included in the sampling frame in each of the three selected localities; the third group was excluded for the study. Afterwards, a circular systematic random sampling was used to select households. If more than one worker belongs to a household, the target respondent was selected using the KISH table [16]. A hundred households were chosen in each of the three areas for each of the two categories, i.e., tannery and non-tannery workers, by the circular systematic random sampling technique. Out of 600 households, a total of 284 households of tannery workers and 289 HHs of non-tannery worker(s) were interviewed successively (Figure 2).

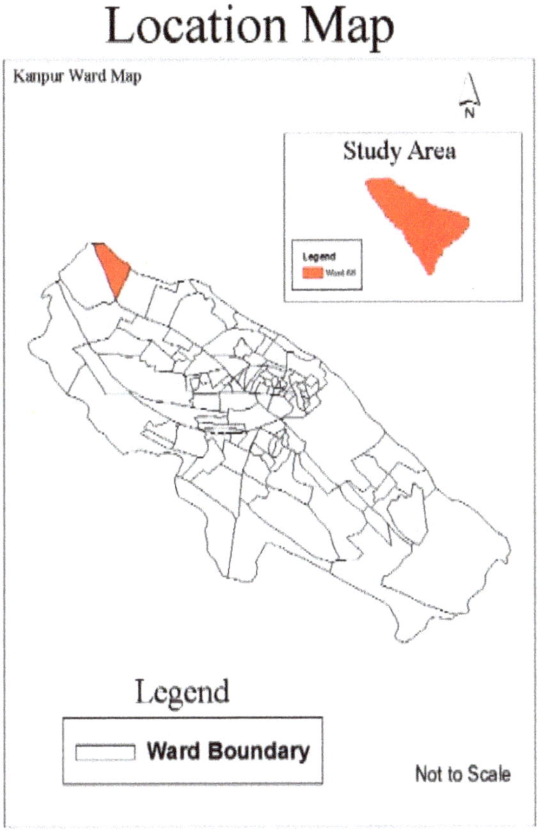

Figure 1. Location map for the study area.

The study is a part of the Ph.D. thesis research work; we have received ethical clearance from the Student Research Ethics Committee of the International Institute for Population Sciences Mumbai, India. We have also obtained consent to participate from each of the respondents before starting the interview.

2.4. Participants and Occupational Categories

The study has covered 284 male tannery and 289 non-tannery age group workers 18–70 years old from the Jajmau area of Kanpur. We have inquired about the respondent's occupation and classified them into two categories: tannery and non-tannery workers.

2.4.1. Dependent Variable

The tannery and non-tannery workers reported symptoms-based prevalence of sinus and nasal allergies. We have considered the following symptoms for nasal allergy (nose full of phlegm and runny, spastic, itchy problems) and sinus (problems such as swelling in your nose, watery nose, phlegm, nose closure) to understand the severity of the health issues.

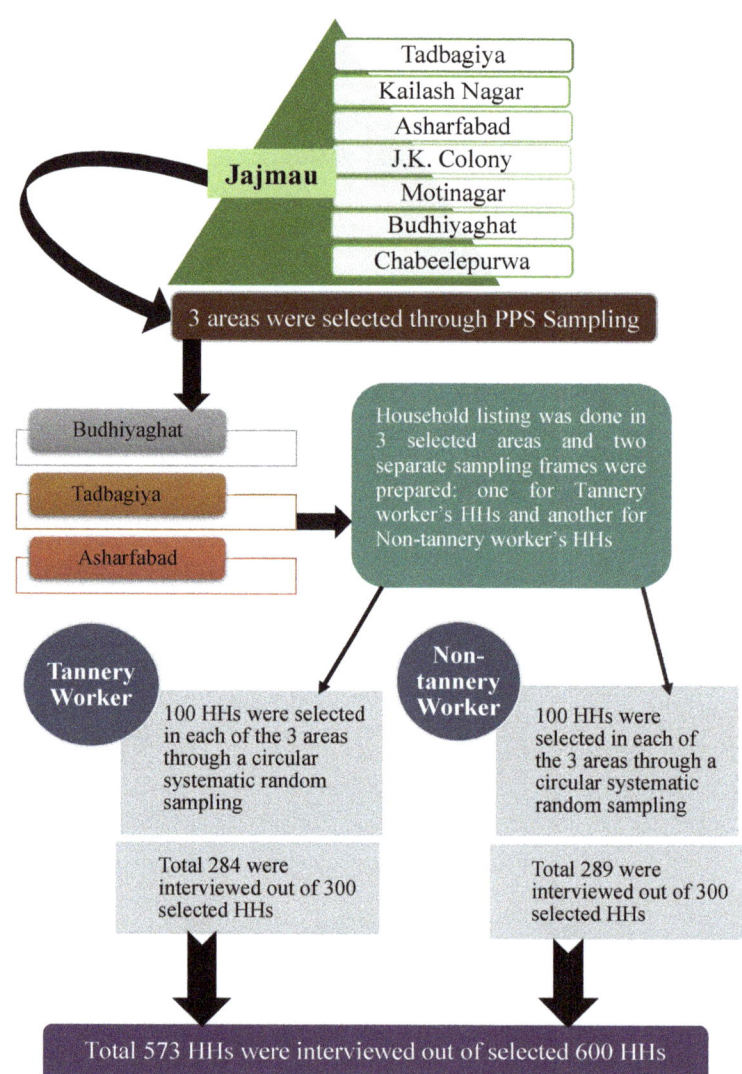

Figure 2. Sampling design for the study.

2.4.2. Independent Variables

Independent variables utilized in this study can be broadly grouped into two categories as socio-economic characteristics or background characteristics and their work-related characteristics. Background characteristics of tannery and non-tannery workers included their age in three category (16–24 years, 25–35 years, and 36+), education in to four category (no education, up to primary, middle school, and higher secondary and above), marital status (currently married, never married, and widowed/widower), religion namely Hindu and Muslim, media exposure (low, medium, high) and their standard of living Index (low, medium, high). The second group of independent variables utilized work-related characteristics of tannery workers, which includes type of job contact (temporary job (daily wages) and permanent job), type of work engagement of tannery workers (beam house work, wet finishing work, dry finishing work, and miscellaneous work), type of work engagement of non-tannery workers (industrial work, manual work, construction work, clerical work, business and shop, and others), work experience in current and previous tannery, and average working in a day and days in a week. Additionally, exposure of chemical in the air (no exposure, low exposure, and moderate/high exposure), airborne dust exposure (no exposure, low exposure, and moderate/high exposure) and headache problems (no headache, up to 10 times, more than 10 times but not every day, and almost every day) have been included in the study.

The qualitative rating of exposure assessment of variables airborne dust and chemical in the air was estimated as follows. The variable airborne dust (no exposure, low exposure, moderate exposure, high exposure, very high exposure) was based on the following qualitative rating of exposure assessment: (0) No exposure: clear visibility. (1) Low exposure: visibility more than 10 m. (2) Moderate exposure: visibility between 5 to 10 m. (3) High exposure: visibility between 1 to 5 m. (4) Very high exposure: visibility less than 1 m. Another important variable, chemicals in the air (no exposure, low exposure, moderate exposure, high exposure, very high exposure), was based on a qualitative rating of exposure assessment as (0) No exposure: no contact with agent; agent is used in workplace but is very unlikely to result in exposure to workers involved. (1) Low exposure: infrequent contact with agent at low concentrations; agent is used in a closed/controlled system; there are no specific activities that enhance exposure; exposure takes place because of presence at the shop floor. (2) Moderate exposure: frequent contact with agent at low concentrations, agent is used throughout the closed/controlled process and exposure mainly occurs by passive contact; infrequent contact is needed with the agent. (3) High exposure: frequent contact with the agent at high concentrations, the nature of the production process and associated manual activities makes regular contact necessary; the agent causes exposure during manual activities and around particular sources such as presses, drums. (4) Very high exposure: frequent contact with the agent at very high concentrations, the agent is used in manual activities that introduce frequent peak exposures such as cleaning, opening a press, spraying paint.

2.5. Data Analysis

Univariate, bivariate, chi-square test, and logistics regression analysis was used to assess the associations between the sinus and nasal allergy with the predictor variables. The odds ratio from the logistic regression analysis was performed by considering the outcome variable as dichotomous (i.e., binary or 0–1), and the predictor variable (work-related characteristics and socio-economic variables) was considered a categorical or a mixture of the two. Results of logistics regression were explained with the help of two different models. Model-1 deals with the socio-economic variables, including (age, education, religion, caste, media exposure, and standard of living index). Moreover, Model-II included work-related variables additional to socio-economic variables. The data entry was done in the CSPro.06 software, and for the data analysis, STATA (Version 13.1) was used.

3. Results

3.1. Demographic and Socio-Economic Characteristics of Tannery and Non-Tannery Workers

Table 1 presents the percentage distribution of selected socio-economic and demographic characteristics. The overall sample of tannery workers and non-tannery workers was 284 and 289, respectively. More than half (54%) of the tannery workers and over three-fifths (63%) of non-tannery workers were age 36 years and above. The majority of the study participants were illiterate, tannery workers (66%), and non-tannery workers (62%). Only 12% of the tannery workers and 20% of non-tannery workers had studied up to high school and more. Two-thirds of tannery workers (66%) are Muslim, and the remaining are Hindus. Furthermore, two-thirds of the tannery workers (66%) belong to the scheduled castes. It indicates that mostly the people from disadvantaged caste groups are engaged in tannery work. Nearby one-fifth of the tannery workers, as well as non-tannery workers, had low levels of media exposure. Further, poverty often reflects a low standard of living and a lack of economic resources.

Table 1. Percent distribution of tannery and non-tannery workers by some selected background characteristics in Kanpur, India, 2015.

Variables	Tannery Workers (%)	Non-Tannery (%)	χ^2-Value
Total	100.0	100.0	
Age in years			
16–24	10.2	6.9	$\chi^2 = 6.007$
25–35	36.3	29.8	$p < 0.050$
36+	53.5	63.3	
Education			
Illiterate	66.1	62.2	
Up to primary	13.4	9.0	$\chi^2 = 9.249$
Middle school	8.8	8.7	$p < 0.026$
High school and above	11.7	20.1	
Marital Status			
Currently married	85.5	89.9	$\chi^2 = 2.629$
Never married	9.4	6.3	$p < 0.269$
Widowed/Widower	5.1	3.8	
Religion			
Hindu	33.8	40.8	$\chi^2 = 3.023$
Muslim	66.2	59.2	$p < 0.082$
Caste			
Schedule caste	65.5	36.3	$\chi^2 = 48.75$
Other backward class	18.3	34.3	$p < 0.000$
Others	16.2	29.4	
Media exposure			
Low	22.9	21.1	$\chi^2 = 0.263$
Medium	48.6	42.2	$p < 0.048$
High	28.5	36.7	
Standard of living index			
Low	37.7	29.2	$\chi2 = 4.673$
Medium	31.3	36.1	$p < 0.097$
High	31.0	34.7	

Standard of living index includes electricity, bed, chair, table, cot, pressure cooker, sewing, machine, Liquid petroleum gas (LPG) gas, mobile phone, water pump, electric fan, color TV, mixer grinder, refrigerator, radio, watch, cycle, motorcycle. Media exposure includes: Newspaper, magazine, movies, TV, radio, and internet.

3.2. Work-Related Characteristics of Tannery and Non-Tannery Workers

The work-related characteristics of tannery and non-tannery workers has been presented in Table 2. The mean age of male tannery workers was 38 years (SD = 1.4). The vast majority of male tannery workers (89%) are working on temporary job contracts, and the rest (11%) are engaged in this occupation on a permanent basis. The respondents work in various tannery processes. A little over 8% are involved in beam house work, 24% are involved in wet finishing, 50% are involved in dry finishing, and 17% are involved in miscellaneous kinds of work. In addition to that, non-tannery workers worked in numerous job categories that are broadly classified into six domains. Around 12% of the non-tannery workers engage in industrial work, while 27% engage in manual work, 20% engage in construction work, 10% engage in clerical work, 25% engage have their own business and shop, and 7% engage in other job categories. The mean duration of their job was 10 (SD = 0.9) years. The average work experience of male tannery workers was 18 years. The male tannery workers also reported that they work almost every day of the week with a 9-h working day as the norm. On average, they worked 6.5 days (SD = 0.6) a week and 9.5 h (SD = 0.2) a day, which is a violation of the labor law according to the factory act in India.

Table 2. Work-related characteristics of tannery workers in Kanpur, India, 2015.

Variables	(%)	(N)
Age in years (Mean ± SD)	38.5 ± 1.4	284
Type of Job contract		
Temporary job (daily wages)	89.1	252
Permanent job	10.8	32
Type of work engagement of tannery workers *		
Beam house work	8.4	24
Wet finishing work	24.2	69
Dry finishing work	50.5	142
Miscellaneous work	16.8	49
Type of work engagement of non-tannery workers **		
Industrial work	11.7	34
Manual work	26.5	76
Construction work	20.0	58
Clerical work	10.0	24
Business and shop	24.5	71
Others	7.0	21
Work experience in current tannery (Mean ± SD)	10.1 ± 0.9	284
Work experience in previous tannery (Mean ± SD)	7.9 ± 1.3	99
Average working hours in day (Mean ± SD)	9.5 ± 0.2	284
Average working days in a week (Mean ± SD)	6.5 ± 0.1	284

* Note: Beam house work: In the beam house, the raw hides processing starts by either stretching the hides on bamboo frames or by pegs, or spreading the hides on the ground in mild sun. Beam house workers frequently come in touch with water and chemicals during preparatory operations such as soaking, liming, fleshing, deliming, bating, and picking. Wet finishing: The wet finishing process includes splitting, shaving, waxing, and oiling. Operations are predominantly performed standing at machines. Dry finishing: Laborers in the dry finishing stage perform operations such as drying, shaving, buffing, pressing, staking, padding, and scraping. Miscellaneous work: There is a group of miscellaneous workers such as packers, sweepers, carriers, and mixers of chemicals. Carriers carry wet hides, and mixing of chemicals is usually done with bare hands. ** Industrial work that includes mechanical workers, small-scale industry workers, repairing workers, furniture workers, hotel workers, mill workers, machine operators, factory workers, manufacturing workers, welding workers, etc. Manual workers include bora handling (bora dhona), rickshaw pullers, horse driving, loading and unloading workers, paining workers, plumbers, etc. Construction workers include raajmishtri, construction labors, contractors, etc. Clerical workers include accountant, clerk, official job, stock in charge, supervisor, computer operators, etc. Business and shop includes those who own their own business, hair cutting shops, thela vendors, electric shops, food shops, fruit sellers, vegetable vendors, Paan shops, general stores, lakdi ka Taal, milk men, scrap businesses, stalls, tailors, tea shops, etc. Others include those in air force jobs, bank jobs, call centers, managers, priests, security guards, drivers, etc. The key issue is that tannery as well as non-tannery workers who belong to the same socio-economic background and live in the same locality have different work exposures.

3.3. Prevalence of Reported Sinus and Nasal Allergies

The prevalence of reported sinus and nasal allergies by some selected background characteristics is presented in Table 3. It was found to be higher among tannery workers aged 36 years and more (15%), while it was 11% among workers in the age group 25–35 years. No significant association of education level with sinus and nasal allergies was observed. About 10% of the workers with a low standard of living index had sinus problems, while it was 14% among those with a high standard of living. Similarly, while looking at nasal allergy, it has been observed that the prevalence of nasal allergy was higher among tannery workers aged 36 years and above (15%) than those in the age group of 16–24 years (6.9%). Prevalence of nasal allergy was higher among workers who had no education (16%) as compared to workers with a middle-school education (8%). A significant difference was found in the prevalence of nasal allergy in Muslim tannery workers (15%) and Hindu ones (7.3%). There was a higher prevalence of nasal allergy among Schedule caste /Schedule tribes (SC/ST) (13%) than others (8.7%). The odds of sinus problems among tannery workers 12 months prior to the survey are presented in Table 4. The model is adjusted for age, education, religion, caste, and standard of living. The results suggest that workers working in tanneries for 6 to 10 years were significantly more likely to develop sinus problems (Odds Ratio (OR)= 3.17; $p < 0.05$) as compared to workers with 5 or less years of engagement in tannery works. Workers with low exposure to airborne dust were significantly more likely to develop sinus problems (OR = 4.16; $p < 0.05$) than those without exposure. When the model is adjusted for age, education, religion, caste and standard of living, years of engagement, type of work and type of job contract, the results suggest that the headaches are significantly more likely to develop nasal problems if they occur almost daily (OR = 1.5; $p < 0.05$) compared to those who had no headaches. Similarly, workers are more likely to develop sinus problem than those suffering from nasal allergy (OR = 20.6; $p < 0.01$) compared to those who were not suffered from nasal allergy.

Table 3. Prevalence of sinus and nasal allergies reported by the tannery and non-tannery workers in Kanpur, India, 2015.

Background Variables	Tannery Workers			Non-Tannery Workers		
	Sinus [%, CI]	Nasal Allergy [%, CI]	Number (N)	Sinus [%, CI]	Nasal Allergy [%, CI]	Number (N)
Age in years						
16–24	13.8 [5.16–32.00]	6.9 [1.67–24.33]	29	0.0 [0.0–0.00]	0.0 [0.0–0.00]	21
25–35	10.7 [5.98–18.35]	9.7 [5.27–17.19]	103	1.2 [0.1–7.93]	4.7 [1.73–11.85]	85
36+	15.1 [10.24–21.80]	15.1 [10.23–21.80]	152	5.5 [2.95–9.89]	7.7 [4.56–12.54]	183
Education						
Illiterate	12.8 [8.72–18.47]	15.5 [10.96–21.47]	187	3.9 [1.86–8.01]	7.8 [4.66–12.81]	179
Up to primary	15.8 [7.16–31.29]	10.5 [3.93–25.24]	38	3.9 [0.05–23.65]	3.9 [0.05–23.65]	26
Middle school	16.0 [5.98–36.30]	8.0 [1.93–27.66]	25	4.0 [0.05–24.45]	8.0 [1.93–27.65]	26
High school and above	12.1 [4.53–28.60]	0.0 [0.00–00.00]	33	3.5 [0.08–12.97]	1.7 [0.02–11.50]	58
Religion						
Hindu	14.6 [8.78–23.22]	7.3 [3.49–14.60]	96	6.8 [3.40–13.04]	5.1 [2.28–10.92]	117
Muslim	12.8 [8.68–18.38]	14.9 [10.45–20.77]	188	1.8 [0.05–5.33]	7.0 [4.01–11.99]	172
Caste						
SC/ST	13.4 [9.22–19.18]	12.9 [8.77–18.57]	186	6.7 [3.1813.40]	5.7 [2.57–12.21]	105
Other backward class	7.7 [2.87–18.99]	13.5 [6.48–25.86]	52	4.0 [1.51–10.36]	7.1 [3.38–14.18]	98
Others	19.6 [10.40–33.75]	8.7 [3.25–21.24]	46	0.0 [0.0–0.00]	3.5 [2.44–13.47]	86
Media exposure						
Low	13.8 [7.30–24.68]	9.2 [4.16–19.22]	65	6.6 [2.45–16.37]	9.8 [4.44–20.38]	61
Medium	11.6 [7.19–18.15]	15.2 [10.10–22.27]	138	4.1 [1.70–9.53]	9.0 [5.03–15.61]	122
High	16.0 [9.49–25.82]	9.9 [4.98–18.64]	81	1.9 [0.04–7.31]	5.3 [0.01–6.49]	106
Standard of living index						
Low	10.3 [5.75–17.69]	11.2 [6.44–18.79]	107	4.7 [1.78–12.11]	8.3 [3.99–16.57]	85
Medium	16.9 [10.37–26.20]	13.5 [7.77–22.36]	89	4.8 [1.99–11.11]	4.8 [1.99–11.11]	104
High	13.6 [7.86–22.60]	12.5 [7.01–21.28]	88	2.0 [0.04–7.73]	6.0 [2.70–12.80]	100
Total	13.4	12.3	284	3.8	6.3	289

Table 4. Odds ratio showing risk factors of sinus problems among tannery workers (12 months preceding the survey) in Kanpur, India, 2015.

Variables	Model-1	C.I.	Model-II	C.I.	Model-III	C.I.
Age in years						
16–24 ®						
25–35	0.90	[0.25–3.22]	0.91	[0.22–3.86]	0.79	[0.16–3.83]
36+	1.40	[0.41–4.83]	1.57	[0.38–6.49]	1.41	[0.30–6.50]
Education						
Illiterate ®						
Up to primary	1.10	[0.39–3.10]	0.87	[0.28–2.68]	1.22	[0.36–4.20]
Middle school	0.81	[0.20–3.20]	0.81	[0.18–3.68]	0.89	[0.14–5.52]
High school and above	0.54	[0.14–2.10]	0.42	[0.09–1.87]	0.74	[0.14–3.87]

Table 4. Cont.

Variables	Model-1	C.I.	Model-II	C.I.	Model-III	C.I.
Religion						
Hindu [R]						
Muslim	0.72	[0.32–1.60]	1.54	[0.60–3.98]	1.49	[0.52–4.27]
Caste						
SC/ST [R]						
Other backward class	0.53	[0.17–1.66]	0.75	[0.21–2.69]	0.76	[0.22–2.57]
Others	1.85	[0.72–4.77]	0.93	[0.31–2.80]	1.18	[0.26–5.42]
Media exposure						
Low [R]						
Medium	0.78	[0.31–2.00]	1.01	[0.36–2.86]	3.04	[0.94–9.78]
High	1.39	[0.42–4.61]	1.55	[0.41–5.86]	2.66	[0.74–9.59]
Standard of living index						
Low [R]						
Medium	2.15 *	[0.87–5.29]	2.45 *	[0.89–6.75]	3.059 *	[0.920–10.16]
High	1.65	[0.61–4.44]	2.17	[0.70–6.71]	2.810	[0.795–9.926]
Work experience in current tannery						
Up to 5 Yrs [R]						
6 to 10 Yrs			3.17 **	[1.17–8.59]	4.46 **	[1.48–13.38]
11+ Yrs			1.64	[0.54–4.96]	1.28	[0.36–4.52]
Type of work						
Beam house work [R]						
Wet finishing work			1.55	[0.28–8.69]	1.64	[0.25–10.83]
Dry finishing work			1.44	[0.27–7.69]	1.31	[0.21–8.06]
Miscellaneous work			0.77	[0.12–5.05]	0.50	[0.06–4.23]
Type of Job contract						
Temporary job (daily wages) [R]						
Permanent job			0.46	[0.12–1.75]	0.28	[0.06–1.38]
Chemicals in the Air						
No exposure [R]						
Low exposure			1.31	[0.41–4.23]	1.05	[0.30–3.66]
Moderate/High exposure			0.39	[0.07–2.37]	0.18 *	[0.02–1.35]
Airborne dust						
No exposure [R]						
Low exposure			4.16 **	[1.22–14.18]	4.69 **	[1.16–18.88]
Moderate/High exposure			1.20	[0.22–6.54]	0.72	[0.11–4.65]
Headache Problem						
No headache [R]						
Up to 10 times					1.28	[0.46–3.56]
More than 10 times but not every day					2.23	[0.51–9.73]
Almost every day					1.52 **	[0.23–9.98]
Nasal Allergy						
No [R]						
Yes					20.59 ***	[6.09–69.63]

Note: [R] Reference category, *** $p < 0.01$, ** $p < 0.05$, * $p < 0$.

4. Discussion

In this study, the self-reported prevalence of nasal allergy and sinus among the tannery workers was considered to understand the severity of the health issues. The primary data were collected and analyzed from one of the major leather tanning industries situated in Kanpur. Tannery workers are exposed to different harmful exposures that include leather dust, chromium dust, and many injurious chemicals [17,18]. The tannery workers frequently come across the dust, which leads to nasal allergy (nose full of phlegm and runny, spastic, itchy problems) and sinus (problems such as swelling in your nose, watery nose, phlegm, nose closure). This study has utilized the qualitative rating of exposure assessment for the two variables airborne dust and chemical in the air to understand its severity.

Results portrays that a large number of people engaged in tannery work are illiterate. A vast majority of the tannery workers were from economically weaker and marginalized sections (schedule caste) of the society. According to Section 38 of Indian Constitution, the principle of the welfare state is accepted to improve the socio-economic conditions of the depressed class of the society. Workers from an unorganized sector are an example of a depressed class in the society, and leather workers are among them. Most of the tannery workers belong to economically and socially backward classes. This class of workers apparently lives a life of poverty, insecurity, and social isolation. The respondents work in various tannery processes such as beam house work, wet finishing, dry finishing, and miscellaneous kinds of work and results cumulate that half of the proportion of the workers is involved in dry finishing.

The male tannery workers reported that they work almost every day of the week with a more than 9-h working day as the norm, and they have been working for a long time, as the average work experience of tannery workers was 18 years. Findings from the study conducted among leather tannery workers in Kanpur reported that the mean age for tannery workers was 34.05 ± 8.96 years and that for non-tannery workers was 32.97 ± 10.59 years ($p = 0.14$), while the tannery workers had a mean duration of work at tanneries for 6.99 ± 4.86 years [19].

Overall, 13.4 and 12.3% prevalence of sinus and nasal allergy has been reported by tannery workers, and higher age group of tannery workers suffered largely. Nasal and sinus allergies are a significantly prevalent occupational hazard among tannery workers, and this study found that the severity increases with the age and the duration of work in the tannery. The other study revealed a significantly higher prevalence of morbidity among the exposed tannery workers in contrast to that observed in the non-tannery (40.1% vs. 19.6%). The respiratory diseases were mainly responsible for a higher morbidity among the exposed workers, whereas the gastrointestinal tract problems were predominant in the control group. The high morbidity among the tannery workers may be due to elevated levels of urinary and blood chromium levels resulting from increased air levels of chromium at the work place. Professional exposure to Cr (III) increases the risk of dermatitis, ulcers, and perforation of the nasal septum and respiratory illnesses as well as increased lung and nasal cancers [7–14].

Workers with low exposure to airborne dust were significantly more likely to develop sinus problem (OR = 4.16; $p < 0.05$) than those without exposure. Dust is produced during several processes in tanning operations: chemical dust can be produced during the loading of hide-tanning drums; and leather dust impregnated with chemicals is produced during some mechanical operations, including buffing [20]. An important health risk factor for the tannery workers is occupational exposure to chromium, which is used as a basic tanning pigment. The workers on exposure to leather dust, which contains chromium in the protein-bound form, exhibited a higher mean concentration of urinary and blood chromium than the reference values [7]. Another study among tannery workers in Bangladesh stated that the prevalence of diseases among the tannery workers is very high and is extremely associated with different working areas of leather processing and the lack of proper PPE (personal protective equipment) use [21].

The results of the study portray that the headaches are significantly more likely to develop nasal problems if they occur almost daily in comparison to those who had no headaches. Similarly, those tannery workers who were suffering from nasal allergy were more prone to develop sinus problem compared to those who did not suffer from nasal allergy. Allergy can cause chronic inflammation of the sinus and mucus linings. Sinusitis is an inflammation of the nasal sinuses, which is commonly caused by bacterial infection following a viral infection such as the common cold. Other risk factors for developing sinusitis include untreated allergies, crooked nasal anatomy, smoking, nasal polyps, and overuse of decongestant nasal sprays. The signs and symptoms of sinusitis vary depending on the level of severity of the inflammation and which sinuses are involved. Headache is one of the primary symptoms of developing nasal allergies to sinus [22].

5. Conclusions

Due to the prolonged exposure to harmful chemicals in tanneries, the workers are prone to nasal allergies, which affect a higher proportion of tannery workers than non-tannery workers. Sinusitis is experienced by a greater proportion of tannery workers than non-tannery ones. Nasal allergies are more prevalent among Muslim and SC/ST tannery workers than their Hindu counterparts. Similarly, a higher prevalence of nasal allergy has been noted for SC/ST workers compared to others. To prevent the many health issues that tannery workers usually experience, we suggest that medical observation, including pre-employment and periodic medical controls, should be performed and must include pulmonary function tests. Improving the overall working condition and ensuring necessary protective regulations for the tannery workers can eliminate many of the environmental exposures that are responsible for these health hazards.

6. Limitations of the Study

- ✓ The use of a cross-sectional survey to collect data may have underestimated the true prevalence of morbidities.
- ✓ The results of self-reported morbidities could be biased due to subjectivity in responses as the severity was not quantified.
- ✓ Recall bias may also have affected the estimated prevalence of morbidities.

Author Contributions: Conceptualization, G.C.K.; Software, S.K.S.; Writing—Original draft, D.V. All authors have read and agreed to the published version of the manuscript.

Funding: This research received no external funding.

Institutional Review Board Statement: The Student Research Ethics Committee (SERC) of International Institute for Population Sciences, Mumbai, India has approved the PhD research.

Informed Consent Statement: Informed consent was obtained from all subjects involved in the study.

Data Availability Statement: This study is based on primary data.

Conflicts of Interest: The authors declare no conflict of interest.

References

1. Heggannavar, A.B.; Harugop, A.S.; Madhale, D.M.; Walavalkar, L.S. A randomised controlled study to evaluate the effectiveness of shortwave diathermy in acute sinusitis. *Int. J. Physiother. Res.* **2017**, *5*, 2066–2072. [CrossRef]
2. Pratibha, M. 1 in 8 Indians Hit by Chronic Sinusitis: Study, TNN, Updated: 11 April 2012. Available online: http://timesofindia.indiatimes.com/articleshow/12615317.cms?utm_source=contentofinterest&utm_medium=text&utm_campaign=cppst (accessed on 16 December 2020).
3. Rosheena, Z. Prone to Sinusitis? Air Pollution in Your City Is Making It Worse. 2018. Available online: https://fit.thequint.com/fit/sinusitis-and-pollution-in-india#gs.X5Jft29n (accessed on 16 December 2020).
4. Ateeq, M.; Hameed, U.; Rehman, S.Z.; Ullah, F.; Khan, A.R.; Zahoor, B.; Akbar, N.U.; Saeed, K. Evaluation of health risks among the workers employed in tannery industry in Pakistan. *J. Entomol. Zool Study* **2016**, *4*, 244–246.
5. Browning, E. *Toxicity of Industrial Metals*, 2nd ed.; Butterworth: London, UK, 1975; Volume 119, pp. 249–260.
6. Walsh, E.N. Chromate hazards in industry. *J. Am. Med. Assoc.* **1953**, *153*, 1305–1308. [PubMed]
7. Rastogi, S.K.; Pandey, A.; Tripathi, S. Occupational health risks among the workers employed in leather tanneries at Kanpur. *Indian J. Occup. Environ. Med.* **2008**, *12*, 132. [CrossRef] [PubMed]
8. Stern, R.M.; Berlin, A.; Fletcher, A. International conference on health hazards and biological effects of welding fumes and gases. *Int. Arch. Occup. Environ. Health* **1986**, *57*, 237–246. [CrossRef]
9. Angerer, J.; Amin, W.; Heinnrich-Ramm, R. Occupational chronic exposure to metals. *Arch. Occup. Environ. Health* **1987**, *59*, 503–512. [CrossRef] [PubMed]
10. Lin, S.C.; Tai, C.C. Nasal septum lesion caused by chromium among chromium electroplating workers. *Am. J. Ind. Med.* **1994**, *26*, 221–228. [CrossRef]
11. Stern, A.H.; Bragt, P.C. Risk assessment of the allergic dermatitis: Potential of environmental exposure to hexavalent chromium. *J. Toxicol. Environ. Health* **1993**, *40*, 613–641. [CrossRef] [PubMed]

12. Mikoczy, Z.; Hagmar, L. Cancer incidence in the Swedish leather tanning industry: Updated findings 1958–99. *Occup. Environ. Med.* **2005**, *62*, 461–464. [CrossRef] [PubMed]
13. Veyalkin, L.V.; Milyutin, A.A. Proportionate cancer mortality among workers in the Belarussian tanning industry. *Am. J. Ind. Med.* **2003**, *44*, 637–642. [CrossRef] [PubMed]
14. Basketter, D.; Horev, L.; Slodovnik, D.; Merimes, S.; Trattner, A.; Ingber, A. Investigation of the threshold for allergic reactivity to chromium. *Contact Dermat.* **2001**, *44*, 70–74. [CrossRef] [PubMed]
15. Rabbani, G.; Billah, B.; Giri, A.; Hossain, S.M.; Mahmud, A.I.; Banu, B.; Ara, U.; Alif, S.M. Factors Associated with Health Complaints Among Leather Tannery Workers in Bangladesh. *Workplace Health Saf.* **2020**, 2165079920936222. [CrossRef] [PubMed]
16. Kish, L. A procedure for objective respondent selection within the household. *J. Am. Stat. Assoc.* **1949**, *44*, 380–387. [CrossRef]
17. Stern, F.B. Mortality among chrome leather tannery workers: An update. *Am. J. Ind. Med.* **2003**, *44*, 197–206. [CrossRef] [PubMed]
18. Kornhauser, C.; Katarzyna, W.; Kazimierz, W.; Malacara, J.M.; Laura, E.N.; Gomez, L.; González, R. Possible adverse effect of chromium in occupational exposure of tannery workers. *Ind. Health* **2002**, *40*, 207–213. [CrossRef] [PubMed]
19. Gupta, R.C.; Ranjan, R.; Kushwaha, R.N.; Khan, P.; Mohan, S. A questionnaire-based survey of dry eye disease among leather tannery workers in Kanpur, India: A case-control study. *Cutan. Ocul. Toxicol.* **2014**, *33*, 265–269. [CrossRef] [PubMed]
20. IARC. Wood, leather and some associated industries. Lyon, 3–10 June 1980. In *IARC Monographs on the Evaluation of the Carcinogenic Risk of Chemicals to Humans*; Distributed for IARC by WHO: Geneva, Switzerland, 1981; Volume 25, pp. 1–379.
21. Hasan, M.; Hosain, S.; Asaduzzaman, A.M.; Haque, M.A.; Roy, U.K. Prevalence of Health Diseases among Bangladeshi Tannery Workers and associated Risk factors with Workplace Investigation. *J. Pollut. Eff. Control.* **2016**, 1–3. [CrossRef]
22. ASCIA (Australian Society of Clinical Emmunology and Allergy). Sinusitis and Allergy. 2015. Available online: https://www.allergy.org.au/patients/allergic-rhinitis-hay-fever-and-sinusitis/sinusitis-and-allergy (accessed on 16 December 2020).

MDPI
St. Alban-Anlage 66
4052 Basel
Switzerland
Tel. +41 61 683 77 34
Fax +41 61 302 89 18
www.mdpi.com

Sinusitis Editorial Office
E-mail: sinusitis@mdpi.com
www.mdpi.com/journal/sinusitis

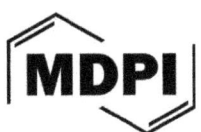

www.ingramcontent.com/pod-product-compliance
Lightning Source LLC
LaVergne TN
LVHW070547100526
838202LV00012B/406